The Role of
the Preceptor

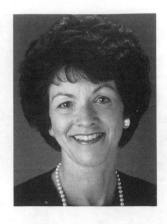

Jean Pieri Flynn, Ed.D., R.N., received her bachelor's degree in nursing from the University of Rochester, Rochester, NY, a master of arts degree in inservice education, a master's degree in medical-surgical nursing and education, and a doctor of education degree in research and nursing administration from Teachers College, Columbia University. Dr. Flynn is currently Director, Home Care Organizational Development at The Mount Sinai Home Health Agency and a health care and management consultant. She has had extensive experience in Staff Development and Continuing Education both as an instructor and as a manager at two large metropolitan teaching hospitals in New York City. She was also a faculty member at Columbia University School of Nursing. Dr. Flynn has been a presenter at numerous national management workshops and research conferences. She is the author of several articles and two books on leadership, medical-surgical nursing and teaching strategies.

The Role of the Preceptor

A Guide for
Nurse Educators and Clinicians

Jean Pieri Flynn
Editor

Springer Publishing Company

Springer Publishing Company, Inc.
536 Broadway
New York, NY 10012–3955

Cover design by Margaret Dunin
Production Editor: Kathleen Kelly

96 97 98 99 00 / 5 4 3 2

Library of Congress Cataloging-in-Publication Data

The role of the preceptor: a guide for nurse educators and
    clinicians / Jean Pieri Flynn, editor
        p.   cm.
    Includes bibliographical references and index.
    ISBN 0-8261-9460-5
    1. Nursing—Study and teaching (Preceptorship)
I. Flynn, Jean Pieri.
[DNLM: 1. Preceptorship—organization & administration.
2. Education, Nursing—organization & administration.
WY 18.5 R744 1997]
RT74.7.R65   1997
610.73'071'55—dc20
DNLM/DLC
for Library of Congress   96-41728
                                                            CIP

Printed in the United States of America

CONTENTS

FOREWORD

All too common are the "war stories" about student clinical experiences and the ineffectiveness of staff education for the neophyte nurse. This book provides an opportunity for reversing a common professional flow. The content focuses on the definition and clarification of the role of the nurse preceptor. Knowledge development surfaces as the constant thread in the establishment of significant professional relationships in clinical practice. The presentation of adult learning theory as a conceptional framework for educative practice and program design is a refreshing departure from the traditional pedagogical approaches. The partnership orientation in the learning paradigm is an important factor that each contributor states or implies. For the student and novice nurse a partnership attitude serves as a seeding for collegial relationships that are so critical in the development of competent nurse practitioners and nurse leaders. The assessment instruments, case studies diagrams and tables stimulate creative thinking. The "step-by-step walk through" in the program designs provides an important meaningful guide for nurse educators.

This book is written for several audiences:

- The student, having no idea about a preceptor arrangement who can learn about the role and its complexities.
- The nurse novice/neophyte who can develop understanding about the parameters of the role, the contractual nature in the preceptor relationship and an appreciation for her responsibility in the partnership dyad.

- Collegiate service sector educators who can refocus how they perceive the preceptor role and clear up the haze that shrouds various elements in the first step of clinical practice for students and novice nurses. This refocusing process can facilitate the restructuring of a significant bridge between academe and the practice world.

- Nurse managers, who have the pivotal function of selecting preceptors and energizing the practice environment. They are challenged to reflect and rethink this responsibility in the patterning of professional nursing.

For all nurses who worry about the positioning of professional nursing in the academic and practice setting, and who struggle with the shaping of health care for the next century, this book provides a giant learning step for the beginning practical phase—the where and when for nurses entering the system for the first time.

ELEANOR BARBA, EdD, MBA, RN

Consultant/Former Dean, School of Nursing, Adelphi University

CONTRIBUTORS

Barbara Stevens Barnum, PhD, RN, FAAN, is a professor at the Columbia University School of Nursing, New York City, and Editor of *Nursing Leadership Forum* at Springer Publishing Company. Prior to these appointments, she was editor of *Nursing & Health Care*, the journal of the National League for Nursing. Dr. Barnum was Director, Division of Health Services, Sciences and Education at Teachers College, Columbia University, also holding the Stewart Chair in the Department of Nursing Education, and, for part of her tenure, the Chairmanship of the Department of Nursing Education.

Anne Elizabeth Belcher, PhD, RN, FAAN, received her bachelor's degree in nursing from the University of North Carolina at Chapel Hill, her master's degree in nursing (medical-surgical nursing education) from the University of Washington, Seattle, and her doctoral degree in higher education from the Florida State University, Tallahassee. Dr. Belcher is currently Associate Professor and Chair, Department of Acute and Long-term Care, at the University of Maryland School of Nursing, Baltimore. She has addressed national and international audiences and has published on topics related in nursing care of the person with cancer, with an emphasis on the psychosocial aspects of the disease. Her previous experiences include Director of Nursing Staff Development at the University of Alabama Hospitals, which implemented a successful internship program for new graduates. Dr. Belcher has also served as mentor to baccalaureate, masters, and doctoral students and faculty in Florida, Alabama, New York, and Maryland.

Janet Mackin, RNC, MS, CNA, received her master's degree in nursing from the Graduate School of Nursing, Pace University, New York City, and a master's degree in adult education from Teachers College, Columbia University, New York City. She is currently a doctoral candidate in the AEGIS Program at Columbia University. She is certified in Nursing Continuing Education/Staff Development and Nursing Administration. Currently, Ms. Mackin is Director of Education and Organizational Development at St. Luke's-Roosevelt Hospital Center in New York City. Ms. Mackin has written and lectured extensively on staff development issues and has been featured in two video programs on self-instructional materials.

Mary Jo Manley, EdD, RN, received her bachelor's degree from Ohio Wesleyan University in Delaware, Ohio, her master's degree in nursing from Yale University School of Nursing in New Haven, CT, and her doctoral degree in higher and adult education from Teachers College, Columbia University, New York City. She is currently Associate Dean in Academic and Clinical Affairs and Assistant Professor in Clinical Nursing at Columbia University School of Nursing. Formerly she was Associate Vice President for Nursing Education, Development and Research at St. Luke's-Roosevelt Hospital Center in New York City. Her clinical background is in mental health / psychiatric nursing and she has practiced as a clinical nurse specialist at New York Hospital-Cornell Medical Center, Westchester Division, and New Jersey Neuropsychiatric Institute, Princeton, New Jersey. In her various positions in both academia and service, she has consistently worked to bridge the gap between education and practice.

Ann M. O'Mara, PhD, RN, received her bachelor's degree in nursing from the State University of New York at Buffalo, her master's degree in nursing from Catholic University, Washington DC, and her doctorate in adult and higher education from the University of Maryland, College Park. Dr. O'Mara is currently an assistant professor at the University of Maryland School of Nursing and coordinates the clinical practicum for senior undergraduate students. Her recent publications are in the areas of rewarding staff nurse preceptors and oncology nursing.

Kathleen V. Studva, MA, RN, received her bachelor's degree in nursing from Hunter College, New York City, and her master's degree in staff development from Teachers College, Columbia University, New York City. She is currently an Education Manager at St. Luke's-Roosevelt Hospital Center, New York City. She has been involved in the development and implementation of preceptor programs throughout her professional career. Her recent presentations, both locally and nationally, address varying aspects of independent study design.

ACKNOWLEDGMENTS

There were several colleagues, family members, and friends who contributed to and facilitated the writing of this book. First, I extend my sincere appreciation to Dr. Ursula Springer at Springer Publishing for the opportunity to work on this book. Special thanks go to Dr. Barbara Barnum for the guidance and support she provided throughout the preparation of the book. I thank Ruth Chasek, Sheri Sussman and Kathleen Kelly at Springer Publishing for their assistance, high standards, and availability throughout the editing process.

To George Flynn, my husband, I extend my loving thanks for his patience, support, and active participation in the preparation of this book. Finally, I thank each of the authors who were hard working and timely in submission of manuscripts, and who provided the expertise so necessary for a book of this nature.

ACKNOWLEDGMENTS

PREFACE

The idea for this book was generated at a colloquium for nurse educators and nurse clinicians. One of the nurse practitioners attending this colloquium said that she liked having students to precept in the clinical setting, but that she had no idea how to plan experiences for these students or how to teach them. This practitioner felt very competent about her knowledge base and about taking care of patients, but she felt inadequate in providing a meaningful clinical experience for students. Although she found several articles about various aspects of precepting in nursing journals, she could locate no book that covered all the essential information.

This book, therefore, is intended as a practical "how to" guide for nursing faculty and for nursing clinicians who want to set up preceptor programs, to guide student experiences, or to help orient novice practitioners to the practice setting.

For those interested in differentiating among precepting, mentoring, and teaching, Chapter 1 describes the parameters. Chapter 2 provides insights into preceptor programs from a standpoint of Adult Learning Theory. Finally, for those interested in programs that go beyond preceptorships, Chapter 5 provides insights into programs such as internships, residencies and mentoring.

Chapter 3 is written primarily for nursing educators and includes a practical example of a preceptor program that has been successfully implemented at The University of Maryland School of Nursing. Chapter 4 is intended primarily for nursing clinicians. In this chapter a highly successful preceptor program for nurse

orientees in a large, urban medical center is described. Both of
these chapters give a clear picture of the advantages of such programs and a practical description of how to implement similar
programs in one's own setting.

Effective preceptor programs do not happen automatically; they
involve careful planning on the part of both preceptor and program
administrator. The hope is that this book will provide a useful
framework for developing and implementing preceptor programs,
for precepting others, and for facilitating the development of nursing expertise in preceptees of all sorts.

— Jean Pieri Flynn,

Editor

Chapter 1

PRECEPTING, NOT MENTORING OR TEACHING: VIVE LA DIFFÉRENCE

Barbara Stevens Barnum, RN, PhD, FAAN

Precepting, of course, is what one defines it to be. In the definition used here, precepting is different from either teaching or mentoring. What the three share is that they are all based on an essential inequality, where one person (teacher, preceptor, mentor) has something to teach that the other, more junior person wants to learn. Although rooted in unequal power, all parties to these relationships may achieve personal and/or professional gains through them.

In order to create generic terms that can be used for all three cases, the senior member in the relationship will be called a *tutor* and the junior member a *pupil*. While these are rather stuffy terms, this allows us to reserve the more common terms for the subsets. *Instructing* will be used generically. Obviously, the use of these terms in this way is simply a convention for the purposes of this chapter.

Teaching, precepting, and mentoring, are three subsets in the instructing relationship, with precepting falling somewhere between teaching and mentoring on the continuum.

Teaching is a relationship in which someone (the teacher) conveys knowledge (about something) to an individual or group of learners (the students). The relationship is primarily one-way,

1

from teacher to student, often with compensating evaluation and corrective measures, and typically some general conversational exchanges for clarity.

In formal courses, the evaluations may take the form of class presentations, tests, papers, or projects receiving feedback. In laboratory courses, there may be individual correction and feedback on experiments, procedures, and various applications. Good teaching probably has more two-way interaction than poor teaching.

Everyone, of course, has had teachers who could hold classes spellbound without students saying a word. And most people have had at least one teacher whom they resented because the students were given an inordinate amount of responsibility for conducting the course, with the teacher adding few additional thoughts or clarifications.

Nor does all teaching take place in the formal setting; it can be on-the-spot and incidental. Head nurses teach staff members every day; staff nurses teach their peers. The impetus in both formal and informal situations is that the junior person or persons needs to learn something.

In the emotive structure of teaching there is little requirement for an intimate or close relationship between the parties. A teacher may be distant to the students or more friendly with some than others. Some teachers become motherly, sisterly, or treat students like buddies, but none of these stances is a requirement for effective teaching.

Teaching is about learning *something*, and is structured around what is to be taught or learned, that is, the content. The personal aspects are secondary.

Mentoring goes to the other extreme of the spectrum. Unlike teaching, which may occur one-to-one or one-to-many, mentoring takes place in a one-to-one relationship. Here a senior person and a more junior person voluntarily enter a relationship whereby the senior both instructs and, more or less, guides the junior career's and career choices over a sustained period of time—often a lifetime.

What gets conveyed in a mentorship cannot be defined in anyone's curriculum. The content addressed changes as the relationship grows and the people change. Essentially, the mentor instructs in or facilitates whatever the junior person needs to learn (in order to get ahead) at any given time. This may involve knowledge, know-how, politics, philosophic stances, introductions to the right people, or finagled invitations to make important presentations. Name it, and it may enter the mentoring relationship at some stage.

A mentorship may even involve nonprofessional lessons, such as how to promote a career while retaining a spouse, or where to find the best tax accountant. In a mentorship, the personal and the professional are beautifully and messily compounded and intermixed.

Mentorships are never the result of an assignment, although they may grow out of a preceptorship or a teaching relationship. They often occur simultaneously, on the basis of some personal spark, when a work situation brings two people together in a superior-subordinate relationship.

Mentoring is the term most nurses prefer when they foster the careers of protégés, partly because they tend to dislike using any terms that are characteristic of the "old boys'" network. Mentoring provides a good two-way interpersonal relationship, in which both parties benefit from the relationship, though, one could argue, the protégé usually *benefits* more and the mentor usually *invests* more.

The main problem with mentoring is that it lacks equivalent terms like tutor/pupil or teacher/student. This chapter uses mentor/protégé, the latter instead of the more awkward term—*mentee*. The term, protégé, carries some of the right-feeling tone for a mentorship. A mentor is personally invested in the success of the protégé. Indeed, the protégé's success is a measure of the mentor's own success. The term *protégé* connotes that sense of advocacy.

In essence, a mentorship is more about the person than about what is taught. The shift is from content to person, from specifics to career development. The emotive structure is important, and the relationship is intimate.

Precepting, in this definition, falls in between teaching and mentoring. Like mentoring, it is a one-to-one relationship. Even if a person precepts more than one student, each relationship tends to be handled in a one-to-one manner. A preceptorship also is sustained over time, but usually a much shorter time than a mentorship: not a lifetime, perhaps a school term, perhaps a year.

While mentorships are formed when something clicks between two people, each of whom has something to bring to the other, preceptorships tend to be contractual or informally arranged. Often they occur between people who did not know each other beforehand. Sometimes there is an interview first, if the relationship is to be on the sustained side or if the senior person is considering a number of candidates. Sometimes apprentices are assigned duties, as when an organization needs someone oriented to a job or role and someone else is assigned to show them the ropes.

The goals of a preceptorship tend to be definite, even when they are broad in context. For example, an experienced head nurse may precept a new head nurse through the experience of learning to run a unit. True, that is a broad goal, but when the purpose and objectives are deemed to be achieved, the preceptorship ends. Nobody precepts someone else through a lifetime.

While it resembles the mentorship in being a one-to-one relationship, the preceptorship is more like teaching in respect to content. There are learning goals to be achieved and they are professional, not personal.

Yes, the preceptorship has a touch of the personal because the evaluation and correction tends to be adjusted on an individual basis. In essence, it is more personal than most teaching, less personal than most mentorships. A preceptorship is more about specific content than a mentorship, but usually about broader, less restrictive content than teaching.

The most difficult thing about a preceptorship is finding an adequate vocabulary to describe it. Teacher/student and mentor/protégé work fine, but preceptor/preceptee? The latter term is very unsatisfactory: too stiff and too derived. For purposes of this chapter, the person who is precepted is labeled an *apprentice*. This term actually fits the relationship quite well. In any domain, an apprentice is there to learn from a master. The experience of the latter and the inexperience of the former sets the type of relationship they will have.

LEARNING CONTEXT

Now that the three basic instructing/learning relationships have been differentiated, the differing contexts in which they occur must be examined, chiefly because the context determines what learning methods will be used. Teaching tends to be the stuff of which classes and conferences are made. Mentoring, on the other hand, is more closely involved with informal on-the-spot education based exclusively on assessment of the protégé's performance on the problem of the moment.

Again, precepting falls in the middle. Some learning situations in a preceptorship may resemble teaching. For example, the apprentice may be given reading assignments, projects, and other materials with which to interact. Often the progress of the apprentice will be judged on these matters, as well as on performance. Nevertheless, of the three forms of instruction, precepting tends to be the one most exclusively related to actual practice performance in a given role.

REIMBURSEMENT

One of the simplest and most pragmatic ways to differentiate among the three tutor-pupil relationships is by looking at the flow of cold hard cash. Simply put, for a sustained or formal relationship, teachers expect to get paid, whether they are faculty or staff development instructors. For incidental teaching, the "payment" may be producing a coworker who no longer asks so many questions. Or, for patient teaching, the payment may be the rewarding sense that the patient will manage satisfactorily when he gets home.

There is not enough money in the world, however, to reimburse a mentor. These are voluntary relationships, given out of the goodness of the mentor's heart. Mentorships are never formal agreements. If they are, they are actually preceptorships. If reimbursement takes place, it may be in the form of personal gifts now and then. And, at least in my experience, the mentor is on the giving end more often here, too. After all, the protégé is likely to be of an age to have weddings, childbirths, and new positions to celebrate. What does the mentor have? Perhaps a retirement if she lives long enough. Mentor rewards exist, of course, but they tend to consist in pride in one's accomplishments.

Once again, preceptorships fall somewhere in between. Some nurses volunteer to be preceptors "out of the kindness of their hearts," but it is a professional kindness rather than a kindness to a particular apprentice. In some organizations preceptors gain status and, in some places, salaries are adjusted to compensate for the added responsibility.

More commonly, an institution receives some reimbursement for providing preceptors for students, though many continue to precept students "for the sake of the coming generation of nurses." This generosity, alas, is fading as the pressures of the present economic crunch in health care grow. Precepting, like other forms of instruction, takes a lot of valuable time.

GENERALIZATIONS AND INSTANTIATIONS

Another difference among teaching, precepting, and mentoring, is that teaching almost always deals with presenting rules, norms, principles, and generalities. One learns for example, the *norms* of anemia, not *how differently the symptoms may appear* from one patient to the next. Teaching is the task of conveying the universals.

Of course, some things really are universal; for example, one should always clear the airway before administering resuscitation. But lots of so-called universals are more tricky. Establishing rapport with a patient may be a good dictate—in most situations—but how one does this will differ radically from one patient to the next, and from one nurse to the next. Rotating weekends equally among staff may be a good principle for any head nurse, but it may not work if one of her staff is in school Mondays and Wednesdays, another is a Seventh Day Adventist, and one party lover considers Friday and Saturday to be the weekend.

Here is where preceptorships and mentorships have a great advantage. If teaching gives the universals, these other forms of education build an appreciation in the learner for the subtleties and varieties (instantiations) that hold forth in the real world. That, incidentally, is where these forms of education take place: in the workplace, not it the classroom (unless one is orienting a student teacher).

ROLE MODELING

The notion of role-modeling brings up another major difference in teaching methods. Precepting and mentoring involve a lot of role-modeling followed by moments of one-to-one reflection on the mentor's/preceptor's performance. Mentoring and precepting may also involve opportunities for the protégé/apprentice to perform under the watchful eye of the senior person, again followed by retrospective analysis or on-the-spot correction, if possible.

Often in role-taking and role modeling, there is a subtle difference between precepting and mentoring. In precepting, the apprentice is known as, and identified as, a learner. In mentoring, that may or may not be the case. For example, a vice president for nursing may serve as a mentor for an assistant vice president, who is not in a student role, but in a subordinate role. Here the junior person is an informal learner, picking up skills, responsibilities, or strategies in preparation for an eventual upward movement. Meanwhile, the protégé holds full job accountability in the institution. The apprentice is rarely a permanent staff person in this sense, and rarely has this sort of accountability in an organizational sense.

NURSING TRADITIONS

For generations *teaching* has been the dominant technique in the education of nurses. Indeed, nurses have gone out of their way to avoid the notion of apprenticeship. Learning on the job (as it was envisioned then) was low-class and nonacademic. It has taken generations to recognize the mistake in overreacting against an apprenticeship model. Indeed, Benner's work (1984) brought home the fact that not everything gets assimilated in a classroom or in one return demonstration.

Indeed, in a complex and dynamic field like nursing, the instantiations may not look much like the schoolroom generalizations at all. In nursing, patients, employees, and bosses do not act like averages, and all the generalizations learned in classrooms may not apply to Patient X in situation Y. And one may go for months or years before meeting the patient with a "normal" heart attack, or an "average" case of diabetes.

Indeed, to find a textbook case of anything is quite astounding. This is why, incidentally, a student who can recite the definition of classic denial may miss identifying such a syndrome in her patient. Benner's expert nurse is one who has been around the instantiations long enough to develop a certain savvy. The expert is accustomed to patients and situations that don't resemble the textbook. She can diagnose and respond to the atypical case, recognizing that of which it is an instantiation. That is why Benner's nurse is not likely to say, "This is a case of denial." She is more likely to say, "Mr. X reminds me of a patient I had last year. He was clever at hiding his denial too."

There are some things that can only be learned by a great deal of experience with a lot of instantiations, hence the need for apprenticeships.

ROLE INCULCATION

Sometimes, a big part of mentoring and precepting is giving the protégé/apprentice a chance to *be* the role, to internalize the role. Just like new grandmothers often protest that they do not "feel" like grandmothers, graduation does not make a nurse feel like a nurse, and promotion does not make a staff nurse feel like a head nurse. New roles, like new robes, have to be worn a while before they fit comfortably.

Teaching is not designed to foster role inculcation, but preceptorships and mentorships can achieve this. That is why people say roles are not taught, but caught.

WHICH MODEL? WHEN AND WHERE?

This is not to say that precepting and mentoring are better than teaching: they are just different. Each form of instructing has its place, and usually one cannot be substituted for the other with much efficiency. Teaching usually comes first. After all, one cannot learn the exceptions unless one knows the rules. For most types of learning, teaching is more efficient than trial-and-error apprenticeship in the work place. So most faculty members, for example, teach a bit about the brain and its potential deficits before turning students loose on a neurological ward.

What formal teaching cannot do is inculcate a role or provide diverse experience. A teacher functioning as a teacher does *not* model staff nurse behavior: she models teacher behavior. Maybe that is why so many new graduates want to be teachers. That is what they have seen if they were "protected" from being close to practicing nurses during their learning experiences.

A role model is someone already doing the job to which the learner aspires, or doing the same job as the learner but doing it more effectively. Here the form of instruction we need is work experience or assisted experience in the form of a preceptorship or mentorship.

Teaching is a cost-effective form of instruction. You can lecture to a group of hundreds as easily as to a group of two. Even the feedback can be mass-managed with objective tests. But one-to-one relationships give a feedback and correction that simply is not available any other way.

Still we see some subtle differences between the preceptorship and the mentorship. The good preceptor may focus on having the apprentice "do it right," in other words, focus on skill acquisition. A skilled mentor, however, is able to ask, What is the best way for this particular protégé, replete with flaws, faults, talents, and opportunities, to achieve?

A WORD ABOUT METHODS

Each form of instruction has methods of conveying information that work, those that work less efficiently, and those that do not work at all. Some of the worst errors in instruction occur when the tutor selects methods that best fit with other systems.

Let us look first at formal teaching, particularly classroom teaching. Here the instructor has a wealth of appropriate methods: lectures (provided they add insight into what the students can learn from reading their assignments); case studies that focus on the "average patient or condition;" directed discussions, provided they are really directed, demonstrations (of normative methods)? and other classical methods. The fancy ones include symposium, debate, case presentation, and problem studies, among others.

While we tend to value classroom teaching more than other methods, the truth is that this is one of the easiest forms of instruction. Any teacher with just a bit of cleverness will soon figure out which classroom methods work best.

Informal teaching is a bit more tricky. Take, for example, the nurse who tries to teach insulin administration and the basics of diabetes care to a newly diagnosed patient. Here the subject matter becomes tough to convey, because emotions get in the way. First, the patient may not have truly accepted the diagnosis yet— even if he thinks he has. The patient who can't quite believe he is a diabetic is working against himself when he tries to "learn" diabetic care.

Additionally, if the patient happens to be ill, the situation adds to the stress. Learning one is diabetic is stressfull enough alone, but if the diabetes is discovered in the wake of a serious imbalance or as part of a surgical work-up for another condition, there is double jeopardy. All the literature on teaching tells us that people are very inefficient learners when they are under stress. Yet, ironically, much of our teaching takes place in the hospital (or other health-care setting) when the patient is under great stress.

The teacher, in this case, must assume that the task will take teaching, reteaching, and lots of corrective feedback. Audio-visuals will be most useful here, as will take home materials that can be reviewed and recycled when the patient is under less stress. The same stress factors, of course, will pertain to a nervous nurse being taught to do parenteral lavage or any other procedure perceived as complex.

Mentoring may require a bit of teaching, but mostly it involves retroactive analysis of the protégé's performance in some situation or on some task. Proactive preparation for the given task may also be needed. Usually the tasks involved here are more complex than nursing procedures. For example, the protégé and mentor might do a retrospective analysis of how the protégé did on running a meeting. They would look at what worked, what did not, and what should be tried the next time. Mentoring sometimes involves bailing out the protégé if he gets in over his head.

Mentoring also may include discussing the mentor's performance on some task, again with proactive or retrospective review. This is the role-modeling aspect. An insightful mentor does not expect the protégé to become a duplicate model, but allows room for differences in style and capabilities.

Another important part of mentoring is promoting the protégé's career. There are numerous ways in which this can be done, from recommending the protégé for progressively more important positions, to opening doors to important people, to helping the protégé solve career-impeding problems.

Just as we do not consider it very good mothering when the 35-year-old single son still lives with his mother, we do not consider it good mentoring when the protégé is kept in eternal servitude, never allowed to fly solo. There are many cases when a protégé has been kept in thrall for too long—for example, someone who has been an assistant to her mentor for 20 years. This is a failed relationship that serves the mentor all too well and stunts the protégé's growth. The ideal is somewhere between *All About Eve* and indentured servitude.

Precepting goes wrong when an insecure preceptor tries to convert precepting into teaching. In this case, the preceptor teaches the apprentice procedures, gives reading assignments, and gives little teaching sessions, but never lets the apprentice get his hands dirty in the real world, where the precepted role takes place. Too much "mothering" or too much protection from the clinical arena (often by withdrawal into conferences) are the errors on one side. Application of the sink-or-swim principle is an error in the opposite direction.

Student Clinical Experience

A Special Case

Student clinical experience is a unique form of learning. While it is often less valued by the institution than classroom teaching or

research, the truth is that it is equally or more difficult to do effectively. A good clinical teacher should be praised and lauded with
honors.

The truth is that good clinical instruction is a blend of a touch of
teaching and a lot of precepting. The teaching part is easy. Indeed,
the new and inexpert clinical teacher is the one who runs around
finding procedures for the students to do. Outside of this, the students are withdrawn from the clinical arena at the slightest excuse.
Why? Because she is more comfortable *teaching*—and the clinical
conference comes closest to that method.

In contrast, the good clinical preceptor immerses the students in
the clinical environment and challenges them to see the irregular-
ities and differences between patients and staff alike. This instructor helps each student consider options when the first one fails. In
this respect, instruction must be individualized. After all, each student is different and each faces a different clinical assignment.

What are the chief ingredients to be found in clinical instruction? There are at least three major responsibilities (beyond
teaching tasks). First, the instructor must spark the student's intellectual curiosity. "Mr. Smith is a lovely shade of brown, but did
you notice, according to the chart, he's Irish? Doesn't that strike
you as curious?"

The next trick is to teach the student to recognize inconsistencies. That is done by presenting problems or things that do not
seem quite right. "Your patient, Mr. Jones, is the funniest most out-
going guy I've ever seen. Here he is, going for a second major
surgery in the morning, and he's joking and laughing with everyone. Most patients would be anxious or scared. What do you think
is going on with Jones?"

The last trick is accurate labeling (one might call this interpretation) of patients who are not typical with appropriate normative
labels. The student who knows the definitions of passive aggres-
sion may mistake it for dependency in Mrs. Doe until she builds a
bit of experience. The good preceptor will help her make a better
fit of labels to patients.

These clinical skills (labeling, spotting inconsistencies, and insa-
tiable curiosity) may or may not be discrete items, but they all have
something to do with forests and trees. The forest is the principle,
the ruling norm; the trees are the instantiations found in patients.

Not every effective tutor will draw rigid boundaries around instruction according to form. However, being aware of the differences among teaching, precepting, and mentoring, may help the instructor make a wiser choice in how to convey information.

SUMMARY

There are at least three basic points on the instruction continuum: teaching, precepting. and mentoring, Each instructional strategy has its own virtues and its own limitations. Together, they uniquely complement each other. Their differences provide a slightly different perspective and serve slightly different goals.

Teaching is content focused, mentoring is student focused. Precepting is also content focused, but the content tends to be broader and of an experiential nature (see Table 1-1).

Experiences with all three sorts of instruction enhance the learning and the career of a nurse. All of these tutor-pupil relationships serve to speed up the learning that occurs by simple immersion in the phenomena (otherwise known as trial-and-error learning, or working for a living).

REFERENCES

Benner, P. (1984). *From novice to expert: Excellence and power in clinical nursing practice.* Menlo Park, CA: Addison-Wesley.

TABLE 1-1 Overview of Teaching, Precepting, and Mentoring

Characteristics	Teaching	Precepting	Mentoring
1. Focus	Content to be taught	Experiential objectives to be achieved	Whatever junior person needs to learn to function in the envisioned role. Focus is on the best way for a protégé to achieve
2. Goals	Professional in nature; not individualized to the learner	Professional in nature; clearly defined	Professional or personal; defined over time
3. Learning Context	Classes/ conferences	Workplace/ performance in the practice setting	Workplace/with informal, on-the-spot education/ feedback
4. Relationship	One-to-many/ one-to-one; usually contractual; ends when content delivered	One-to-one; contractual; time limits set at the start	One-to-one; relationship sustained over indefinite period of time
5. Content	Rules, norms, principles, generalizations	Subtleties and varieties in real-world applications	Adapting one's own style and talents to real world applications
6. Student role	Identified as a learner	Identified as experienced learner	May be identified as skilled learner or as subordinate
7. Evaluation	By tests, papers, projects, presentations	Assessment of individual performance; may include projects	Retroactive analysis of individual performance
8. Reimbursement	Teacher paid, tuitions/fees	Varies from payment to volunteer post	Seldom involves exchange of monies

Chapter 2

ADULT LEARNING CONCEPTS IMPORTANT TO PRECEPTING

Mary Jo Manley, EdD, RN

The discipline of adult education has been evolving rapidly over the last twenty years, with a great deal being written on the subject (Brookfield, 1986, 1987; Brundage & Mackeracher, 1980; Cross, 1981; Kidd, 1973; Knowles, 1988; Knox, 1981; Long, 1982; Lovell, 1980; Mezirow, 1990; Smith, 1982; Tough, 1978; Weathersby & Tarule, 1980). Much of this work has major implications for the teaching/learning of nursing students and staff, all of whom are chronologically "adult." Nurse educators, whether they be teachers, preceptors, or mentors, must understand the importance of applying the concepts of this discipline to the profession of nursing.

This chapter will help you to:

- identify the five domains of adult education;
- identify nine principles of adult learning;
- relate the nine principles of adult learning to effective adult education practice, as it pertains to precepting nursing students or staff; and
- identify your own strengths and weaknesses within each domain and its associated principles.

The literature in adult education centers around five major domains (Manley, 1987): facilitator/preceptor, learner/apprentice, learning environment, learning content, and learning process. A discussion of each domain follows, beginning with facilitator/preceptor.

FACILITATOR/PRECEPTOR DOMAIN

Adult education literature describes the role of the teacher/preceptor as one of facilitator. In the traditional teacher-centered approach to learning, the teacher transmits knowledge to the learner. In the adult education, learner-centered approach, the teacher is a resource who helps learning occur. Thus, the adult education, learner-centered approach puts a completely different emphasis on the learning process. The onus is put on the apprentice to learn. The preceptor cannot "make" the apprentice learn. She can only "facilitate" the learning. Proceeding with this thought, the following principles pertain to effective learning facilitation of nursing students or staff when one is in the role of preceptor. Table 2-1 illustrates the domains of adult education and associated principles of adult learning. Table 2-2 Illustrates how the principles relate to effective adult education practice, specifically precepting of nursing students or staff.

> **PRINCIPLE 1:** Learning is facilitated when the preceptor has sufficient experience and expertise within an identified clinical practice area to feel confident and competent in nursing clinical practice skills.

This is probably the easiest principle to attain. Preceptors are usually selected or volunteer for the role because they have the experience and practice skills necessary to act as a role model for an apprentice nurse entering clinical service. Generally, preceptors feel confident in their level of skill practice. This is as it should be, for the preceptor is the "master" practitioner and the apprentice is there to learn these skills. In some ways, the preceptor is in the most advantageous position to facilitate nursing education. Apprentices are usually very eager to learn the skills of the preceptor; that is why they entered nursing, to be able to "practice" it. They have great respect for experienced nurses who practice competently. Apprentices come ready to learn, but they cannot just absorb what preceptors already know. The question for preceptors becomes, "How best can I work together with a less experienced nurse or student to help her acquire these same skills with which I feel so comfortable?" To help apprentices learn practice skills, preceptors must do more than practice nursing competently. This brings us to Principle 2.

TABLE 2-1   Domains of Adult Education and
Associated Principles of Adult Learning

Domain	Principles
Facilitator/Preceptor	1. Learning is facilitated when the preceptor has sufficient experience and expertise within an identified clinical practice area to feel confident and competent in nursing clinical skills.
	2. Learners prefer and can learn best from preceptors who understand and appreciate learning, and continue to be learners themselves.
	3. Learning is enhanced by preceptors who demonstrate accurate empathy, non-possessive warmth, respect for the learner, and consistency in their own approach to the preceptor/learner relationship.
Learner/Apprentice	4. Each learner is unique, and one's learning is effected by one's cur rent status in the continua of Physiological/Aging Phenomena; Sociocultural/Life Phases; and Psychological/Developmental Stages.

continued

TABLE 2-1   *continued*

Domain	Principles
	5. Learners learn best if they are full partners in the learning experience, participating fully in the design, implementation, and evaluation of the experience.
Learning Environment	6. The environment that is most effective in enhancing learning has available learning resources.
	7. The environment that most enhances learning is one that is supportive; is free from threat; encourages openness, inquiry, and trust; and avoids competitive judgments of performance.
Learning Content	8. Learning content that is most effective is relevant, useful and clearly organized around exploration of problems perceived as significant by the learner.
Learning Process	9. Learning is most significant when the full, holistic learning process is utilized, which includes: the differentiation, specification, and analysis of thoughts, words, perceptions, actions, and feelings experienced by the learner in a given situation in order to determine meanings, explore significance, and gain fresh new insights; validation, integration, synthesis, and incorporation through usage; and finally back into the system of the learner resulting in growth, authenticity and self-direction.

TABLE 2-2 Principles of Adult Learning Related to Effective Adult Education Practice

Principle	Effective Adult Education Practice
1. Learning is facilitated when the preceptor has sufficient experience and expertise within an identified clinical practice area to feel confident and competent in nursing clinical skills.	• Preceptor is a "master" practitioner. Apprentice is there to learn skills. • Preceptor's role is to facilitate the learning of nursing practice skills by the apprentice.
2. Learners prefer and can learn best from preceptors who understand and appreciate learning, and continue to be learners themselves.	• Preceptor makes an effort to learn about the skills of learning. • Preceptor reflects upon her own learning needs and makes efforts to meet those needs.
3. Learning is enhanced by preceptors who demonstrate accurate empathy, non-possessive warmth, respect for the learner, and consistency in their own approach to the preceptor/learner relationship.	• Preceptor recalls what it is like to learn complex skills for the first time. • Preceptor actively listens and observes apprentice to ascertain where that person is coming from and then communicates understandings back to that person for validation. • Preceptor is warm, open, caring, supportive, and approachable when working with learners without being overly possessive or smothering. • Preceptor demonstrates acceptance of the apprentice and recognition of her as a less experienced colleague.

continued

TABLE 2-2 *continued*

Principle	Effective Adult Education Practice
	• Preceptor is genuine and consistent when working with learners and demonstrates congruence in her words, actions and feelings.
4. Each learner is unique, and one's learning is effected by one's current status in the continua of physiological/aging phenomena; socio-cultural/life phases; and psychological/developmental stages.	• Preceptor takes physiological and aging factors into consideration when planning learning experiences. • Preceptor takes cultural values and views of life into consideration when planning learning experiences. • Preceptor plays an important role in helping the apprentice grow and mature in the "practice" of nursing.
5. Learners learn best if they are full partners in the learning experience, participating fully in the design, implementation and evaluation of the experience.	• Preceptor invites full participation of the learner in the design, implementation, and evaluation of learning experiences.
6. The environment that is most effective in enhancing learning has available learning resources.	• Preceptor helps the learner consult other clinical experts and utilize alternative learning resources (libraries, audio-visual aids) to supplement learning.
7. The environment that most enhances learning is one that is supportive; is free from threat; encourages openness, inquiry and trust; and avoids competitive judgments of performance.	• Preceptor creates a supportive, non-threatening environment that fosters free raising of questions by the apprentices.

Principle	Effective Adult Education Practice
8. Learning content that is most effective is relevant, useful and clearly organized around exploration of problems perceived as significant by the learner.	• Preceptor helps learner develop and grow in problem-solving and decision-making skills within the framework of the immediate unit, patient care assignments, and responsibilities.
9. Learning is most significant when the full, holistic learning process is utilized, which includes: the differentiation, specification, and analysis of thoughts, words,perceptions, actions, and feelings experienced by the learnerin a given situation in order to determine meanings, explore significance and gain fresh new insights; validation through usage; and finally integration, synthesis, and incorporation back into the system of the learner resulting in growth, authenticity, and self-direction.	• Preceptor is consciously engaged in the holistic learning process. • Preceptor encourages the apprentice to become fully engaged in the holistic learning process. • Preceptor aims to provide meaningful learning experiences by understanding the nine adult education principles, completing self assessments for each domain, and then, based upon the results, deciding what follow-up actions need to be taken.

PRINCIPLE 2: Learners prefer and can learn best from preceptors who understand and appreciate learning, and continue to be learners themselves.

This principle points to the preceptor making an effort herself to learn about learning. How does one learn? What does it entail? How do I do it? How do others do it? An effective preceptor reflects upon one's own growth and development, assesses one's own learning needs in light of one's strengths and weaknesses, and then makes efforts to meet those needs. A preceptor who understands learning, who knows how to learn herself, can utilize this knowledge to help the apprentice acquire knowledge and skill in the most efficient, effective manner, with the least amount of pain for the learner, and least burden for the preceptor. In fact, the precepting experience can become a fulfilling and rewarding experience for both parties involved. Both can grow in the experience. Educators are well aware of the old saying that, in a learning experience, the teacher learns far more than the pupil. Because this is an important principle, each domain section in this chapter will end with a preceptor self-assessment so that readers can assess their own learning needs for each domain and its associated principles, and decide what actions they wish to take in response.

PRINCIPLE 3: Learning is enhanced by preceptors who demonstrate accurate empathy, non-possessive warmth, respect for the learner, and consistency in their own approach to the preceptor-apprentice relationship.

Accurate empathy refers to the ability to walk in the learner's shoes, to reach into one's own memories and recall what it was like to be new on a unit, trying to learn complex skills for the first time. Having empathy entails the ability to actively listen to the words and to observe the actions of the apprentice, to ascertain where that person is coming from, and then to communicate observations back to that person in a way that the other knows the first understands. Communicating one's understanding in a way that is verified by the learner makes the empathy "accurate." Suppose, for instance, that, after talking with a new apprentice on the unit a preceptor notices that she was talking very rapidly, fidgeting with her blouse, and glancing about apprehensively. The preceptor might say, "I notice you seem somewhat apprehensive. It's scary going onto a unit for the first time, especially when you are a new graduate and haven't had a chance to become confident in your skills yet." If the preceptor is accurate, chances are she will hear the learner heave a sigh of relief that her anxiety has been recognized in a supportive way. The apprentice will probably begin talking about her concerns, and start feeling more comfortable. As the apprentice becomes more comfortable, the focus can be more fully on learning. If the preceptor is not accurate, the apprentice will tell her so, and may even begin to talk about whatever it is that is bothering her.

Non-possessive warmth refers to being warm, open, caring, supportive, and approachable when working with the learner, without being overly possessive or smothering. Apprentices need to feel comfortable asking questions; they need to know the preceptor will be there if they need her, but they also need to develop independence, skill, and confidence. Independence, skill, and confidence comes gradually. In the interim, in order to assure safe patient care as well as meaningful educational experiences for the apprentice, the preceptor needs to be sure the learner knows what to do and how to do it. One way to do this is to have the apprentice work with the preceptor and observe her in action, but watching and doing are two very different psychomotor skills. When an apprentice is doing a skill for the first time, the preceptor might observe her in action, assist if necessary, and then discuss performance afterwards. Another way to ascertain her ability or skill level is to ask questions. "You have Ms. Green today. How will you go about changing that dressing?" Questions, when put in a nonthreatening, nonjudgmental way, stimulate thinking, create an inquiring environment and foster learning. Asking questions is perhaps one of the easiest and most effective methods of teaching/precepting. In all these instances, if the preceptor is warm and approachable, the apprentice will not hesitate to seek advice and will welcome the preceptor's presence. If, on the other hand, the preceptor is cold and gives the impression of being too busy to have time for the apprentice, the learner may not seek help when needed, or will not ask a question that could enhance her knowledge base. At best, this slows down or deprives the learner from developing confidence and competence. At worse, it could result in unsafe practice.

Respect for the learner is another important interpersonal skill shared by effective preceptors. Each of us is a unique, important individual. The apprentice brings uniqueness to the preceptor-apprentice relationship, coming from a particular background, from a particular culture, from a specific educational situation, and with a variety of experiences. In some ways, being warm, open, and supportive demonstrates respect, but, in addition, adults like to be treated as adults. Apprentice learners are adults, and want to be recognized and respected as colleagues, new to the service, but nonetheless important and equal human beings with ideas and opinions of their own. Respect means valuing the learner as a person and demonstrating positive regard toward that learner.

Consistency of words, actions, and feelings in the preceptor's relationship with the apprentice fosters stability, security, and confidence in the learner. The learner knows what to expect, gets clear and consistent messages as to her progress, and is able to learn more freely and rapidly. Take, for example, the apprentice who is consistently late to the unit and arrives late again saying in an embarrassed manner, "Gosh, I'm sorry about being late again. My alarm clock didn't go off and I overslept. I hope I didn't inconvenience you." The preceptor can acknowledge irritation in a constructive manner by responding, "I have to admit I'm feeling irritated with you. I don't like having these feelings, but waiting week after week for you is frustrating. More importantly, though, I'm concerned about what's happening to you. When you are late, our time together is shortened and you are no closer to the goals you have set for becoming a responsible practitioner. We need to talk about what is happening here." This response acknowledges the preceptor's irritation while still focusing on the learning goals of the apprentice. The preceptor is genuine but empathic. She confronts the apprentice with the realities of the situation in a way that helps the apprentice to see personal inconsistencies and learning barriers, thus giving the opportunity to learn from the experience.

The items identified in Principle 3 are interpersonal skills known as *helping skills*. Research has shown that these are not just something certain people have and others do not, but rather they are truly skills that can be taught and learned (Carkhull, 1969; Hammond et al., 1977). Effective preceptors are nurses who have learned these skills and can demonstrate them as they work with

TABLE 2-3 Self-Assessment: Facilitator/Preceptor Domain

Directions: Circle the appropriate response:

	1–2 years	2–3 year	3–4 years	4–5 years	5+ years
1. My experience within my current practice area is:	Novice	Advanced Beginner	Competent	Proficient	Expert
2. My skill expertise within my current practice area is:					
	To a Very Little Extent	To a Little Extent	To Some Extent	To a Great Extent	To a Very Great Extent
3. I value learning.	1	2	3	4	5
4. I consider myself a learner.	1	2	3	4	5
5. I demonstrate accurate empathy.	1	2	3	4	5
6. I demonstrate nonpossessive warmth.	1	2	3	4	5
7. I respect learners.	1	2	3	4	5
8. I am consistent in my words, actions and feeling.	1	2	3	4	5

Actions to be taken in response to the facilitator/preceptor self-assessment their assigned apprentices. A self-assessment tool for evaluating one's skills within the facilitator/preceptor domain is presented in Table 2–3.

LEARNER/APPRENTICE DOMAIN

The second domain is that of learner/apprentice. Adult education focuses on the learner, rather than on the teacher, and many in the field consider the learner/apprentice domain to be the most important. Without the learner, there would be no need for a preceptor. We are all learners at times and, as was said earlier, in the preceptor–apprentice relationship both parties learn; however, the apprentice is there for the express purpose of learning, and the preceptor is there for the express purpose of helping that apprentice learn. For this interaction to happen most effectively, the preceptor must understand the following principles.

> PRINCIPLE 4: Each learner is unique, and one's learning is effected by one's current status in the continua of physiological/aging phenomena; sociocultural/life phases; and psychological/developmental stages (Cross, 1981).

Traditionally nurses learn that "the patient is a person," unique, whole, and affected by a unique and diverse set of physical, sociocultural, and psychological variables. The same is true of learners, which should not be a surprise, since a great deal of what patients do is to learn. In fact, we are all learners a great deal of the time, so what holds true for learners relates to all of us. Apprentices are unique, come from a variety of backgrounds, learn in a variety of ways, and have a rich diversity of physical, sociocultural, and psychological experiences upon which to build.

Physiological/Aging Phenomena

One's status in the continua of the physiological/aging phenomena can play an important part in learning, and the effective preceptor takes that into account. One must be rested, well-nourished, feeling well, and not under a great deal of stress, to learn best. To focus on the task, to have accurate eye-hand coordination, and to be highly motivated is difficult if one is overly tired, hungry, under great stress, or not feeling well. In addition, reaction time, the speed of learning, and the rapidity of speech as it relates to understanding are different with different people and can change with age. When precepting a staff nurse who has been in the Labor and Delivery area for 30 years and is now being transferred to a rapidly moving step-down unit, the preceptor might expect a different kind and possibly a different rate of learning than that typical of a young, highly motivated new graduate who has chosen to work on the step down unit in order to gain skills that will improve her career, and who feels lucky to have been given the opportunity to work there.

Sociocultural/Life Phases

The above example also illustrates how sociocultural/life phases impact on learning. The new nurse who is just embarking on a new career is at a very different phase in life than the older nurse, who has been in one specialty area most of her life, and now must change specialties at a time when she needs the job to finish putting her children through college. Nurses in their 20s and 30s are looking at different life tasks, and so have different learning priorities than those in their late 40s and early 50s. The former look at long-range goals and career opportunities. They seek order and stability as they are just starting their careers and are searching for anchors. The latter are more apt to be looking back at their choices, accepting their competencies, and feeling less competitive. Such characteristics affect a learner's readiness to assimilate new things.

We all come from a particular cultural background that professes its own particular values and views of life. An apprentice from a cultural background that values obedience and non-assertiveness will learn very differently than someone from a sociocultural system that values assertiveness and questions authority and rules. The preceptor would have to consistently question and carefully listen and watch to understand what the former learner understood or needed to learn. With the latter learner, the preceptor would know readily what the learner was thinking, and would be answering questions and providing rationales for actions. In fact, when preceptors, like the former learner, value obedience, they might even become angry or threatened by such questions.

Most nurses continue to be women. Though times are changing, the socialization of most women encourages strong feelings of duty, commitment, and selfless caring for others, while the socialization of men encourages competition, achievement, and aggressiveness (Bernard, 1981). Preceptors, both for their own self-growth, and for facilitating apprentice learning, need to become cognizant of, knowledgeable in, and sensitive to the new and growing body of knowledge surrounding women's and men's developmental and sociocultural issues as these impact upon learning. By recognizing and expressing one's own gender values, reflecting upon and valuing one's own experiences, preceptors and learners can more fully integrate their thinking, feeling, and doing, thereby becoming a more consistent, whole human being. This is what learning is all about.

Psychological/Developmental Stages

Finally, psychological/developmental stages play a part in learning. How the learner perceives herself in her own psychological development and maturity will impact the way she thinks and the kinds of decisions and judgments she makes. The preceptor's role is to help the apprentice grow and mature in the "practice" of nursing. Asking questions helps the learner reflect on what she is doing and why. "What made you decide to go to that staff nurse to seek help?" "Why do you say you think this patient needs no PRN medication for pain now?" Questions, asked supportively, challenge the learner to think through her decisions, to articulate what she is doing and why, to reflect on her own experience, and to understand herself and her knowledge more clearly for the next decision. Telling her what to do and how to do it does not stimulate this kind of full self-reflective learning. Asking questions portrays to the learner the value and importance of her own experience in her learning process, helping her to grow and mature in the "practice" of nursing, as well as in her own learning skills.

Each person, preceptor, and apprentice, brings her own sociocultural, physical, and psychological background to the learning experience, and to the interrelationship of the two people, which ultimately impacts on the learning that occurs. Preceptors who rec-ognize what they are bringing to the relationship in this regard and who are sensitive to what the learner brings, will be better pre-pared to share their own expertise with the apprentice, thus facili-tating growth and learning in the practice of nursing.

> **PRINCIPLE 5:** Learners learn best if they are full partners in the learning experience, participating fully in the design, implementa-tion, and evaluation of the experience.

Most apprentice learning meets part of this principle. Preceptors and apprentices become actively involved in hands-on caring for patients. Direct patient care is the implementation phase of the learning experience; however, this principle also calls for involving the learner in the design and evaluation of the experience. After all, if each person's experience is unique, then the learning required to best build on this experience is unique. One of the ben-efits of being a preceptor is that the preceptor deals one-on-one with the apprentice, helping her to reflect upon her experience, to assess what learning is needed and, based on that reflection and assessment, helping her attain the experience. This does not mean that the preceptor refrains from identifying important things to be learned. Rather preceptor and apprentice collaborate with each other, contributing to the design of the total learning experience.

For instance, most people know how they learn best. Some need to read first, then hear, then see, then do. Others like to see first, then do, then hear, and then read. Others want someone with them several times when they do a new procedure before doing it alone. Still others feel comfortable doing a new procedure after being coached once. The preceptor's role is to help the learner identify how best she learns, then, using her own judgment and expertise in the practice of nursing, decide how the two can implement a safe approach together.

Participation in the evaluation of the experience is a critical part of the apprentice's learning. This includes both formative evalua-tion, namely, that which is ongoing throughout the experience, and summative evaluation, which occurs as a summary at the end of the experience. In both cases, the preceptor can help the appren-tice reflect upon what happened, analyze the experience, identify

TABLE 2-4   Self-Assessment: Learner/Apprentice Domain

Directions: Circle the appropriate response:

	To a Very Little Extent	To a Little Extent	To Some Extent	To a Great Extent	To a Very Great Extent
1. I am cognizant of my own unique physiological characteristics that impact learning, including:					
State of fatigue	1	2	3	4	5
State of health	1	2	3	4	5
Rate of learning	1	2	3	4	5
Reaction time	1	2	3	4	5
Rapidity of speech	1	2	3	4	5
Tone of speech	1	2	3	4	5
Seeing	1	2	3	4	5
Hearing	1	2	3	4	5
Other	1	2	3	4	5
2. I am cognizant of the apprentice's unique physiological characteristics that impact learning, including:					
State of fatigue	1	2	3	4	5
State of health	1	2	3	4	5
Rate of learning	1	2	3	4	5

Reaction time	1	2	3	4	5
Rapidity of speech	1	2	3	4	5
Tone of speech	1	2	3	4	5
Seeing	1	2	3	4	5
Hearing	1	2	3	4	5
Other	1	2	3	4	5

3. I have reflected upon my own sociocultural/life phase status as it relates to learning, including:

My current life task priorities	1	2	3	4	5
My assumptions about learning	1	2	3	4	5
My assumptions about being a nurse	1	2	3	4	5
My major sociocultural values	1	2	3	4	5

4. I have reflected upon my psychological/developmental stage as it impacts learning, including:

My current developmental stage	1	2	3	4	5
How I perceive myself	1	2	3	4	5
How others perceive me	1	2	3	4	5
How I would like to be perceived	1	2	3	4	5

continued

TABLE 2-4 *continued*

	1	2	3	4	5
5. I learn by reading	1	2	3	4	5
6. I learn by hearing	1	2	3	4	5
7. I learn by watching	1	2	3	4	5
8. I learn by doing	1	2	3	4	5
9. My apprentice learns by:					
Reading	1	2	3	4	5
Hearing	1	2	3	4	5
Watching	1	2	3	4	5
Doing	1	2	3	4	5
10. When I precept, I include the apprentice in:					
Designing the experience	1	2	3	4	5
Implementing the experience	1	2	3	4	5
Evaluating the experience	1	2	3	4	5

Actions to be taken in response to the learner/apprentice self-assessment:

the effectiveness of what occurred and decide how to move on
from there. When learners are involved and participate in all aspects
of the learning process, they become more motivated and committed
to learning. A self-assessment tool for evaluating the learner/
apprentice domain is presented in Table 2-4.

LEARNING ENVIRONMENT DOMAIN

Much has been written on the importance of the environment as it
effects learners, both positively and negatively (Brookfield, 1986,
1987; Friere, 1990; Illich, 1972; Knowles, 1988; Knox, 1977; Mezirow,
1990; Senge, 1987). Most agree with the following principles:

> **PRINCIPLE 6:** The environment that is most effective in enhancing
> learning has available learning resources.

This principle is self-evident, but nonetheless very important.
Research has shown that many nurses perceive "resources" to mean
people. People, of course, are very important resources. The preceptor becomes the primary people resource for the apprentice, but
others on the unit also have expertise to contribute. Apprentices
are often very good at identifying people resources themselves
and in seeking out those persons from whom they feel they can
learn. The preceptor needs to facilitate this process and might ask
herself, "What expertise do others on this unit have? How might
they be utilized to help this apprentice learn?" Arranging for the
apprentice to attend rounds and/or case conferences that relate to
her current activity is often useful.

In addition to people, many health environments have libraries,
audio-visual aids and learning centers. The preceptor needs to be
knowledgeable about those learning resources that are available to
assist with and/or supplement the apprentice's clinical learning.

> **PRINCIPLE 7:** The environment that most enhances learning is one
> that is supportive; free from threat; encourages openness, inquiry
> and trust; and avoids competitive judgments of performance.

This principle goes hand-in-hand with the three principles relating
to the facilitator/preceptor domain. The learning environment of

the apprentice is greatly affected by the qualities of the preceptor. If the preceptor creates a supportive, non-threatening environment that is open to inquiry and free from pejorative judgments of performance, the environment will enhance learning. Others on the unit, head nurse to all the staff nurses, licensed practical nurses, technical assistants, housekeepers, receptionists, physicians, social workers and other health care workers impact the unit's environment and can enhance or impede the apprentice's learning process.

Assessing one's unit in relation to Principle 7 and assessing where the preceptor has some control over the factors identified can be important. If the preceptor is aware of these factors, he or she will be able to maximize this principle whenever possible and to assist the apprentice through situations where others are not interested or knowledgeable.

In addition, if an apprentice finds that a situation is threatening, judgmental, nonsupportive, or closed to inquiry and openness, the preceptor can help the apprentice identify what is occurring, reflect on the experience as it is happening, and look for ways to deal with it. When this occurs, an apprentice can turn a negative experience that hinders learning into one that fosters growth and maturity in the practice of nursing to the fullest extent. After all, the real world is not always supportive. This is an opportunity to identify what is happening now, to find constructive, alternative ways to resolve it and, thus, to be more prepared for dealing with similar events that might occur in the future.

Some institutions have an effective learning environment, as described in Principle 7. Others do not. Literature in many fields, including both adult education and nursing, are focusing on the importance of the environment and its ability to enhance or inhibit learning. Some authors are beginning to suggest that, of the five domains discussed in this chapter, the learning environment may be the most important in its influence on learning (Chopoorian, 1986; Kleffel, 1991; Mezirow, 1990; Senge, 1990). A tool for assessing the environmental domain can be seen in (Table 2-5).

TABLE 2-5 Self-Assessment: Learning Environment Domain

Directions: Complete the following:

1. I have assessed the learning resources available to me and to an apprentice as follows:

People: _____

_____

_____

Books/pamphlets/written material: _____

_____

_____

Hardware (includes overhead projectors, slide projectors, VCR, monitors, etc.)

_____

_____

Computers: _____

_____

Software (includes films, slides, interactive video computer programs, etc.)

_____

_____

Other: _____

_____

_____

	To a Very Little Extent	To a Little Extent	To a Moderate Extent	To a Great Extent	To a Very Great Extent
2. I have assessed my environment and found it to:					
Be supportive	1	2	3	4	5
Be non-threatening	1	2	3	4	5
Encourage openness	1	2	3	4	5
Encourage inquiry	1	2	3	4	5
Encourage trust	1	2	3	4	5
Avoid competitive	1	2	3	4	5

judgments of
performance

continued

TABLE 2-5   *continued*

Actions to be taken in response to the learning environment domain self-assessment:

_____

_____

_____

_____

_____

_____

_____

_____

_____

LEARNING CONTENT DOMAIN

The content domain is often perceived as being of primary importance. In actuality, the content itself may be less important in the
facilitation of learning than the way it is presented, the people
involved, and the context within which it is learned, namely, the
learning environment. Most adult education literature would
agree with the following principle.

> **PRINCIPLE 8:** Learning content that is most effective is relevant,
> useful, and clearly organized around exploration of problems per-
> ceived as significant by the learner.

Certainly, the preceptor-apprentice learning model fits a good
part of this principle. The practice of nursing is the content that the
apprentice is there to learn. It is clearly relevant, useful, and perceived significant by the learner! This is the goal. The preceptor
needs do little to ensure this aspect of the principle. It is this very
content that motivates the apprentice to learn.

The apprentice has now come to the real world, where the problems are real problems. The job now is to learn how to deal with
those problems, and the preceptor's role is to help accomplish that.
For the preceptor, the question becomes how to clearly organize

the content around the exploration of problems. This ties into earlier principles, which spoke to asking questions and providing an environment of inquiry. Adult education consistently points to the importance of helping learners think through situations, reflect upon them, and develop knowledge and skill in the process of problem identification and resolution. This means preceptors will be most effective if they help apprentices develop and grow in problem-solving and decision-making skills within the framework of their immediate unit, patient care assignments, and responsibilities.

Obviously there is no one right way to do this; however, the process involves helping the apprentice identify patient problems, think about ways to address them, take safe effective action(s), and then evaluate the results. It is really helping the apprentice apply the nursing process to increasing numbers of patients until she has significant experience with enough variety of patient symptoms, situations, and responses to practice confidently and proficiently. Benner's (1994) work on how nurses learn to move from novice to expert is a meaningful reference for all preceptors. The preceptor's role in this process is significant, for the preceptor has accomplished the move from novice to competent, or proficient, or even expert. The apprentice recognizes and respects this experience and wants to be independent herself. The preceptor can help speed this learning process by asking questions that help the apprentice reflect and begin to tie together the many pieces of information that must be absorbed. "What did Mrs. Green's skin look like when we gave her the IV for dehydration?" "Does Mr. Smith look like that now?" "Do you think he might be having the same problem or a different one?" "What could you do to determine this?" Questions stimulate inquiry, encourage reflection, and help learners tie together pieces of information for themselves in meaningful, useful ways.

Apprentices need experience dealing with a variety of patient symptoms, situations, and responses in order to incorporate a large enough "bank of experiences" (what Benner [1984] calls *instantiations;* see Chapter 1) within themselves to help them recognize and compare the symptoms, situations, and responses of individual patients. This guides apprentices in their practice, helping them to move from novice to advanced beginner, and on to competent practitioner. Preceptors can help apprentices do this by

helping them to recognize the instantiations, by asking questions
that stimulate reflection about past cases, and by linking them to
current ones. The case presentation approach also helps apprentices reflect on current cases and how they relate to past cases they
have experienced. Anything that helps the apprentice compare the
similarities and differences between patient's situations, symptoms, and responses, helps to build this "bank of experiences."
Table 2-6 presents a tool for assessing the learning content domain.

TABLE 2-6   Self-Assessment: Learning Content Domain

Directions: Circle the appropriate response:

	To a Very Little Extent	To a Little Extent	To a Moderate Extent	To a Great Extent	To a Very Great Extent
1. The content to be learned by the apprentice is:					
Relevant	1	2	3	4	5
Useful	1	2	3	4	5
Clearly organized around the exploration of problems	1	2	3	4	5
2. I ask questions to help the apprentice reflect on similarities and differences between patient situations, symptoms and responses.	1	2	3	4	5
3. I ask questions to help the apprentice identify problems, particularly patient problems.	1	2	3	4	5

	To a Very Little Extent	To a Little Extent	To a Moderate Extent	To a Great Extent	To a Very Great Extent
4. I help the apprentice consider alternative ways to deal with identified problems, particularly patient problems.	1	2	3	4	5
5. I help the apprentice to take safe, effective and appropriate action(s) to address the identified problem(s).	1	2	3	4	5
6. I ask questions to help the apprentice evaluate the results of the actions s/he takes.	1	2	3	4	5

Actions to be taken in response to the learning content domain self-assessment:

_____

_____

_____

_____

_____

_____

_____

_____

_____

_____

_____

_____

_____

LEARNING PROCESS DOMAIN

There are many ways to conceptualize and describe the learning process. According to Brundage and Mackeracher (1980), there seems to be agreement in the literature on four basic steps that are involved in each learning activity. These steps are illustrated in Figure 2.1.

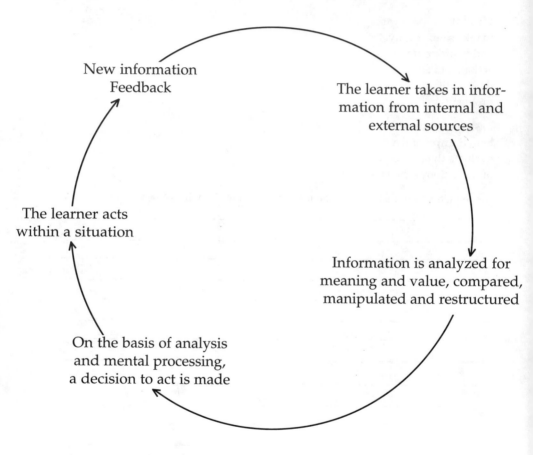

FIGURE 2.1

The process shown in Figure 2.1 can be fully conscious, fully unconscious, or a mixture of both. All of the principles that have been discussed in this chapter affect this process. The feedback portion of this loop is subject to distortion both from outside and within the learner. When feedback is immediate, its potential for modifying learning is enhanced. Analysis for meaning and value is primarily in relationship to personal meaning and value relevant to the learner. This process is cyclical and dynamic, and one enters or ends the process at any point. If the process is not fully implemented, gets thwarted along the way, or the feedback is distorted, learning can be thwarted, impeded, and growth does not proceed. The following principle, based upon this process, reflects current thinking in adult education.

> **PRINCIPLE 9:** Learning is most significant when the full, holistic learning process is utilized, which includes the differentiation, specification, and analysis of: thoughts, words, perceptions, actions, and feelings experienced by the learner in a given situation in order to determine meanings, explore significance, and gain fresh new insights; validation through usage; and finally integration, synthesis, and incorporation back into the system of the learner resulting in growth, authenticity, and self-direction.

This seems to be a long and wordy principle. One needs to read it several times to get a feel for the full conceptualization of a holistic learning model. Learning incorporates the learners cognitive, affective, and psychomotor involvement. The process itself involves pulling apart information, feelings, and actions to specify, compare, and analyze them in order to find one's own meaning and significance; trying out or practicing new insights to see how they work for that learner; and reincorporating the new knowledge back into one's own person, resulting in personal and professional growth, authenticity, and self-direction. Adult literature refers to this holistic process by a variety of terms, such as *praxis* (Friere, 1990), *conscientization* (Friere, 1990), *transformational learning* (Mesirow, 1990), *critical reflectivity* (Brookfield, 1987), *experiential learning* (Peplau, 1957), *reflection in action* (Schon, 1987) or *emancipatory learning* (Apps, 1985). Full implementation of this process results in change, growth, and a more fully functioning human being.

Such learning is not a linear process. Cognitive, affective, and psychomotor domains all interact together with emphasis at any point on one or another, depending upon the apprentice, the preceptor, the environment, the content, or any combination thereof. For the learner, the process is one of differentiation/specification and integration/synthesis, which unfolds new insights and knowledge that is incorporated into the system of the learner, synthesized, and reintegrated into practice.

Brookfield (1985) describes this cyclical learning process as:

Praxis is at the heart of adult education; participants are involved in a constant process of activity, reflection on activity, new activity, collaborative analysis of activity, new activity, further reflection and collaborative analysis and so on. "Activity" can, of course, include cognitive activity so that adult education does not always require participants to do something in the sense of performing clearly observable acts. Exploring a wholly new way of interpreting one's work, personal relationships or political allegiances, would be examples or activities in this sense (p. 48).

This learning process is very congruent with an article published years ago in the *American Journal of Nursing*, and written by Hildegard Peplau (1954), a highly regarded nurse theorist. In this article, Peplau described steps involved in a holistic process of helping students learn. Perhaps adult education and nursing are just now catching up to her! How does the preceptor facilitate this holistic learning process within the learner? One way is by understanding the nine adult education principles outlined in this chapter, assessing one's own strengths and weaknesses as related to each principle, and then deciding what actions to take to follow-up on the assessment results. Fully incorporating the learning process one's self will foster growth and authenticity, which, in turn, will help another learn. Table 2-7 includes a self-assessment tool for the learning process domain.

TABLE 2-7   Self-Assessment: Learning Process Domain

Directions: Complete the following:

		To a Very Little Extent	To a Little Extent	To a Moderate Extent	To a Great Extent	To a Very Great Extent
1.	I understand Principle 9.	1	2	3	4	5
2.	I consciously practice Principle 9.	1	2	3	4	5
3.	I help the apprentice to understand Principle 9.	1	2	3	4	5
4.	I help the apprentice to practice Principle 9.	1	2	3	4	5

Actions to be taken in response to the learning process self-assessment:

_____

_____

_____

_____

_____

_____

_____

_____

Complete the final summary question:

1. The five domains of adult education are:

a) _____

b) _____

c) _____

d) _____

e) _____

_____

_____

SUMMARY

This chapter identified the five domains of adult education. Within those five domains, nine principles of adult learning were discussed. The nine principles were related to effective adult education practice, specifically that of precepting nursing students or staff. A self-assessment tool for each domain and its corresponding principles was provided so that the reader could assess his or her strengths and weaknesses and build action plans accordingly.

REFERENCES

Apps, J. W. (1985). *Improving practice in continuing education: Modern approaches for understanding the field and determining priorities.* San Francisco: Jossey-Bass.

Benner, P. (1984). *From novice to expert: Excellence and power in clinical nursing practice.* Menlo Park, CA: Addison-Wesley.

Bernard, J. (1981). *The female world.* New York: Free Press, Macmillan.

Brookfield, S. (1985, Fall). A Critical Definition of Adult Education. *Adult Education Quarterly, 36(1),* 44–49.

Brookfield, S. (1986). *Understanding and facilitating adult learning.* San Francisco: Jossey-Bass.

Brookfield, S. (1987). *Developing critical thinkers.* San Francisco: Jossey-Bass.

Brundage, D. H. & Mackeracher, D. (1980). *Adult learning principles and their application to program planning.* Ontario, Canada: Research Project under contract by Ministry of Education.

Carkhuff, R. (1969). *Helping and human relations: A primer for lay and professional helpers,* Vol. I (Selection and Training) and Vol. II (Practice and Research). New York: Holt, Rinehart and Winston.

Chopoorian, T. J. (1986). Reconceptualizing the environment. In P. Moccia (Ed.), *New approaches to theory development* (pp. 39–54). New York: National League for Nursing.

Cross, P. K. (1981). *Adults as learners.* San Francisco: Jossey-Bass.

Freire, P. (1990). *Pedagogy of the oppressed.* New York: Herder and Herder.

Hammond, D. C., Hepworth, D. H., & Smith, V. G. (1977). *Improving therapeutic communications.* San Francisco: Jossey-Bass.

Illich, I. (1972). *De schooling society.* New York: Harper and Row.

Kidd, J. R. (1973). *How adults learn.* Chicago: Associate Press, Follett.

Kleffel, D. (1991, Sept.). Rethinking the environment as a domain of nursing knowledge. *Advances in Nursing Science, 14(1),* 40–51.

Knowles, M. S. (1988). *The modern practice of adult education: From pedagogy to andragogy.* Chicago: Follett.

Knox, A. B. (1977). *Adult development and learning.* San Francisco: Jossey-Bass.

Kolb, D. (1981). Learning styles and disciplinary differences. In A. W. Chickering and Associates (Eds.), *The modern American college.* (pp. 232–255). San Francisco: Jossey-Bass.

Long, H. (1982). *Adult learning.* New York: Cambrige University.

Lovell, R. B. (1980). *Adult learning.* London: Halsted.

Manley, M. J. (1986). *Nursing staff development and adult education in a major metropolitan hospital: 1950–1980.* Ann Arbor, MI: UMI Dissertation Information Service.

Mezirow, J. & Associates. (1990). *Fostering critical reflection in adulthood: A guide to transformative and emancipatory learning.* San Francisco: Jossey-Bass.

Peplau, H. (1957, July). What is experiential teaching? *American Journal of Nursing. 57,* 884–886.

Schon, D. (1987). *Educating the reflective practitioner.* San Francisco: Jossey-Bass.

Senge, P. (1990). *The fifth discipline: The art and practice of the learning organization.* New York: Doubleday.

Smith, R. (1982). *Learning how to learn: Applied theory for adults.* New York: Cambridge, The Adult Education Company.

Tough, A. (1978). Major learning efforts: Recent research and future directions. *Adult Education, 28(4),* 250–263.

Weathersby, R., & Tarule, J. (1980). *Adult development: Implications for higher learning.* Washington, DC: American Association for Higher Education.

SUGGESTED READINGS

Brookfield, S. (1995). *Becoming a Critically Reflective Teacher.* San Francisco: Jossey-Bass.

Knowles, M. (1992). *The Adult Learner: A Neglected Species.* (4th ed.) Houston: Gulf.

Liebermax, A., & Miller, L. (eds.) (1991). *Staff development for Education in the 1990s: New Demands, New Realities, New Perspectives.* New York: Teachers College Press.

Mac Gregor, J. (1993). *Student Self-Evaluation: Fostering Reflective Learning,* No. 56. San Francisco: Jossey-Bass.

Chapter 3

A MODEL PRECEPTOR PROGRAM FOR STUDENT NURSES

Ann M. O'Mara, PhD, RN

Nursing schools across the country are implementing innovative clinical courses in response to the many changes occurring in the health care field. Until recently, the traditional approach to clinical teaching was one instructor supervising a group of 8–10 students. This approach creates a number of problems, including (a) inadequate preparation of the student for the real world of nursing; (b) insufficient time to practice complex technologies; and (c) an exposure to the complexities of the particular unit/facility that is superficial and unrealistic. A number of nursing schools have discovered that this artificial reality ignores the immense contributions that experienced staff nurses can make to the student's full realization of nursing practice. Consequently, several nursing programs are utilizing staff nurses as preceptors to help mitigate the reality shock often felt by the new graduate.

PURPOSE

The purpose of this chapter is to:

1. describe preceptorships and the advantages and disadvantages of precepting undergraduate nursing students;

2. describe the roles and responsibilities of the involved individuals;

3. identify important factors in the selection process of faculty and preceptors;

4. describe the process of developing and implementing a preceptor course with reference to a model program; and

5. describe the process for designing and implementing a precepted course with reference to a model program.

PRECEPTOR PROGRAMS IN UNDERGRADUATE TEACHING

Definition

Goldenberg (1987/1988) defines a preceptorship as a one-to-one relationship between an experienced nurse and a neophyte. The process can begin at any time, starting as early as the student's first clinical exposure to the professional role or starting as late as the new graduate's first professional nursing position.

Often preceptorships are confused with apprenticeships, conjuring up in our minds the old diploma programs of the nineteenth century. Imbedded in the old concept of apprenticeship was the notion of contributing to the work environment with learning as a secondary outcome. With preceptorships, learning is and must be maintained as the primary goal. Accomplishing this goal involves a minimum of three individuals—the faculty member, the student, and the preceptor. The remainder of this chapter will utilize this simple triad as the exemplar for discussing all aspects of precepting.

While apprenticeships have a long and troubled history in nursing education, preceptorships are receiving positive evaluations in the contemporary world of nursing education. As early as 1981, Chickerella and Lutz maintained that the advantages of preceptorships outweighed the disadvantages. Just what are these advantages and disadvantages?

Advantages of Preceptor Programs to the Faculty

Sometimes the "price" of a preceptor is that faculty assist in research or continuing staff education. Collaboration in such activities is not only an advantage to the faculty, but may also serve as a reward to the preceptors. With the increased emphasis being placed on scholarly productivity in the academic world, access to patient populations for research is becoming more important and problematic. However, the access problem may be mitigated by the close working relationship that develops between faculty and preceptors. One outcome of this relationship can be the encouragement of staff by faculty to identify researchable clinical problems and ultimately to engage in the research process collaboratively.

In comparison to a few years ago, many staff can no longer enjoy the luxury of attending continuing education courses outside their own facility. Declining resources have also resulted in reduced professional development staff formerly available to provide individualized continuing education programs to the clinical staff. Faculty are well prepared to assist in the preparation and presentation of relevant clinical topics.

Advantages of Preceptor Programs to the Preceptor

A number of advantages and sources of satisfaction have been identified in the literature. In fact, these sources of satisfaction have often been the impetus for clinical agencies to seek collaborative relationships, in the form of preceptorships, with schools of nursing. The most notable advantage is that of increased job satisfaction. Related to this general feeling of satisfaction is the fact that preceptors find that teaching students:

1. adds a new dimension to their work worlds;
2. affords different kinds of teaching opportunities;
3. motivates them to maintain and upgrade clinical skills and knowledge; and
4. results in their learning from students.

In addition to the advantages for the preceptor, there are also advantages for nursing service/education as well. Since the student's performance can be closely scrutinized, recruiting new graduates takes on a different dimension. Nurse managers recognize that orientation of new graduates who have precepted on their assigned units is accomplished more efficiently and effectively.

Advantages of Preceptor Programs to the Student

In general, nursing educators agree that using preceptorships in nursing education, particularly in the student's final semester, can build student confidence, increase the level of independent functioning, provide opportunities for role socialization, and provide opportunities for acquisition of competence and confidence in performing clinical skills (Scales, Alverson, & Harder, 1993; Scheetz, 1989).

On a more practical level, students find their learning needs are more easily met, their anxieties reduced and, most recently, they have a way to demonstrate their skills and knowledge to potential employers. To have their eyes opened to the reality of professional nursing practice is a maturing experience for most. Such comments as, "I had no idea nursing was so multi-faceted," "Nursing is more teamwork than I thought," and "What I was taught in class really is relevant!" demonstrate the tremendous growth nursing students undergo when precepted.

Disadvantages of Preceptor Programs to the Faculty

The evaluation process can produce a number of anxieties for faculty. The preceptor's incomplete or vague information describing student behaviors can create an adversarial relationship with both the preceptor and student.

Instead of the usual one-to-nine student ratio, faculty are now dealing with a preceptor for every student. Site visits and follow-up phone calls to preceptors and students are very time consuming.

In general, the academic term defines the beginning and the ending to courses. Unfortunately, this may not be the case with precepted courses. Several weeks to a month prior to the beginning of the course, faculty must spend a considerable amount of time negotiating student placements and orienting preceptors.

Despite the identified disadvantages to all members of the relationship, preceptorships in undergraduate nursing programs are flourishing. While most programs are utilizing preceptors to bridge the ideal of the educational environment with the reality of the workplace, one program has used preceptorships in its foundational course (Donius, 1988). In this chapter, the focus will be on preceptorships used in the student's final semester.

Disadvantages to the Preceptor

Balancing the needs of the patients with the learning needs of the student is the major disadvantage to the preceptor. This balancing act usually translates into extra time spent and increased responsibility at work. Unfortunately, release time from usual patient assignments for this activity is seldom an option, and preceptors must determine how they will blend patient care with student teaching. For some, this is a challenging and satisfying art and, for others a source of real frustration. Inadequate preparation and inexperienced staff (fewer than 18 months experience) are additional difficulties encountered in using preceptors.

Disadvantages of Preceptor Programs to the Student

In contrast to the profusion of literature on the advantages to the student in a precepted course, there is a paucity of information regarding disadvantages. Goldenberg (1987/1988) identified the evaluation process, preceptee-preceptor relationship, and preceptor absences as causes of student dissatisfaction with preceptorships.

Evaluation Process

Students find the evaluation process more difficult than the usual clinical grading process, particularly those who are in danger of failing. Instead of the usual faculty-student relationship governing the evaluation process, now there is a third person (preceptor) involved in the relationship. Faculty seldom directly observe student behaviors but rely on the preceptors' observations and, based on these observations, faculty judge the students' abilities or inabilities to accomplish the clinical objectives.

Preceptee-Preceptor Relationship

Work expectations and communication styles may be a source of friction in the relationship. What the preceptor expects the student to accomplish and learn may be different from the student's expectations or even beyond the student's capabilities. A quiet, reflective member of the relationship may have trouble relating to a direct, confrontational member.

Preceptor Absences

There are times, due to illness or other commitments, when the preceptor will be absent and another staff member must be the preceptor. Just as students find it hard to rotate from one clinical site to another, similar anxieties and uncertainties arise when the preceptor is absent. This is particularly true when the preceptee-preceptor relationship is a strong, mutually rewarding one.

ROLES AND RESPONSIBILITIES: FACULTY, PRECEPTORS, STUDENTS

The potential success of any precepted relationship relies on a clear understanding of the roles and responsibilities of all involved individuals. The following discussion will highlight the major responsibilities of each member.

Faculty Role

The multiple roles of the faculty in a precepted experience include facilitating the relationships between preceptors and students, monitoring student learning experiences, and evaluating student performance. Of these three, facilitation is the most critical as it requires faculty to be clear and open communicators. Validation, rephrasing, and summarizing conversations with preceptors should be used frequently. When discussing the clinically weak student with the preceptor, faculty may find follow-up, formal written summaries to be the norm. Successful facilitation of the relationships will aid in faculty monitoring and evaluation of student progress.

Facilitation

The work of Hseih and Knowles (1990) summarizes the relevant issues related to the faculty role in facilitating the preceptorship relationship and ultimately monitoring and evaluating students. They identified seven themes as important to the preceptorship relationship:

1. Faculty are the catalysts for building and maintaining *trust* with preceptors and students, as well as between student and preceptor.

2. *By clearly defining expectations of all participants* faculty can greatly reduce confusion among participants. Printed materials in the form of handouts, course description, and a preceptor manual are helpful in reiterating expectations.

3. The usual set of *support systems* are no longer in place for either the preceptor (co-workers often are not preceptors) or the student (peers who may not be on the same unit). The faculty's role is encouraging preceptors and students to verbalize their concerns, problems, and the changed roles associated with preceptorships.

4. Just as all students do not come with all the prerequisite skills and knowledge, not all preceptors possess the requisite teaching and communication skills. *Honestly communicating* the potential for less than a perfect performance to both the preceptor and student sets the stage for a positive experience. By implementing this approach early in the relationship, faculty can avoid the pitfalls inherent in 3-person interactions.

5. The manner in which one learns must be *respected and accepted.* The classic counter example of this principle is the strict and regimented training of our earlier schools of nursing in comparison to the present approach utilizing adult learning principles. Faculty must take the lead in helping the student understand a

preceptor's teaching methodology and, conversely, helping the preceptor understand a student's approach to learning. The goal is to reach consensus and not threaten one's basic personality.

6. Acknowledging feelings of uncertainty and anxiety on the part of both the preceptor and student will go a long way in maintaining everyone's sense of self-worth. Such techniques as self-disclosure, positive feedback, and an attitude of confidence will facilitate an environment of *encouragement*.

7. Faculty successful in implementing the above mentioned aspects of a preceptor program, will require a considerable amount of *mutual sharing of self and experience* between preceptor and student. Closely related to this is the sense of trust that faculty must convey to preceptor and student.

Evaluation of Students

Evaluating student performance is never delegated. Only faculty have the requisite skills and knowledge of the evaluation process for deciding student achievement of course objectives. Emphasizing that this responsibility remains with the faculty can considerably reduce a preceptor's anxiety. On more than one occasion a preceptor has said, "I don't want the responsibility of deciding this student's fate." In reality, the preceptor does play a large role in the decision-making process; however, the final decision and communicating that decision to the student rests with the faculty.

Two issues regarding evaluating students are described as follows:

1. How does one convince the preceptor that faculty determine the student's grade?

In contrast to clinical objectives which are incremental in nature (A, B, C, D, or F), Pass/Fail clinical objectives provide clearer guidelines for identifying student behaviors (preceptor responsibility) and evaluating student performance (faculty responsibility).

From the initial meetings with preceptors, faculty must continually reiterate the preceptor's role in describing student behaviors. The next step involves giving feedback to the preceptor as to faculty interpretation of student behaviors. For example, when a preceptor is unsure as to the safety of a student's actions (using correct techniques, stating accurate rationale), faculty must obtain specific clinical examples, including a time frame, and explain to the preceptor how these actions are (or are not) meeting clinical objectives. Some clinical areas, such as the Intensive Care Unit (ICU), may create in the preceptor's mind a higher expectation of students, thus setting them up for failure. Consequently, considerable faculty guidance of both the preceptor's expectations and the student's preparation is essential. Student anxieties, coupled with the complex medical and emotional patient problems of the ICU, can create a devastating scenario for the preceptor. Faculty should give concrete examples of how the experience should progress from the first clinical day to the last clinical day.

Finally, ongoing, open communication is essential. Asking preceptors about the complexity of the student's patient assignments, how the student prepares, and the student's essential knowledge base will provide a wealth of information as to the student's performance.

2. How does one handle those students who are unsafe, lack adequate knowledge or act unprofessionally?

It goes without saying that some students will not be successful, be it in a traditional or in a precepted clinical experience. When such situations arise, before concluding that the student is not successfully meeting the objectives, faculty must closely scrutinize the setting (including the preceptor). Situation 3-1 illustrates this point.

Situation 3-1
"I had no idea I was anxious"

Students in the precepted course have the opportunity to rank-order the clinical offerings: general medicine-surgery, Intensive Care Unit (ICU), gerontology, ambulatory clinics, perioperative, rehabilitation, pediatrics, maternal-child, mental health, and community health. Given the large class size, faculty are unable to honor all first choices. However, in the case of Laura, her first choice for an ICU was honored.

Her preceptor, in addition to being experienced, was a warm, nurturing individual who would bend over backwards to help students be successful. She recognized the complexities of the ICU and was able to provide rich learning experiences. On the faculty's first visit to the unit, all the non-verbal behaviors of frustration on the part of the preceptor were observed; however, the level of acuity in the unit pre-cluded any in-depth discussion with the preceptor. Laura, on the other hand, appeared calm as she followed the preceptor everywhere.

The faculty's follow-up conversation revealed a disturbing situation. While Laura's nonverbal behavior indicated calm-ness, her conversations with the preceptor and other staff members suggested otherwise. For example, on a particular-ly busy day when one staff member had called in sick, Laura insisted on going to lunch and belittled the staff for not doing the same. When the preceptor reminded Laura of how busy the unit was and how potentially unsafe it could be, Laura responded that she had not thought of it that way. On sever-al occasions, Laura was late arriving, or asked to go home early. Despite the preceptor's and the faculty's spelling out for Laura the inappropriateness of her behavior, it continued.

At the conclusion of the fifth clinical day, with eight more remaining, the preceptor could see no significant improve-ment in Laura's professional demeanor and believed she could no longer be an effective preceptor to this student. Given that this student had no previous record of such behav-ior, the faculty considered other factors, namely, the nature of the intensive care unit. The faculty called Laura into her office, reviewed the sequence of events, and told her she was removing her from this particular setting. In exploring the environment and Laura's desire to be placed in the ICU, two issues emerged. The motivation to work in the ICU was not entirely Laura's. However, she felt compelled to follow the trend of her peers. Many of her friends praised the ICU because "there is much more there to learn." In the final analysis, Laura really thought there was an equal amount to be gained by working on a general medical-surgical unit.

The ICU setting also posed unforeseen problems for Laura. This particular ICU was located in the cancer center of the medical facility. Less than a year ago, Laura had lost her father to acute leukemia, watching him succumb to the complications of sepsis and respiratory failure. During her latest five days in the ICU, the majority of patients were being treated for one or both of these medical problems. In exploring these aspects, the faculty posed the idea that perhaps she had considerable anxiety. At first Laura denied her feelings, but later recognized that her insomnia and loss of appetite might also be related.

Laura was placed on a step-down coronary care unit with the understanding that, without significant improvement in her professional behavior, she would fail the course. By the third clinical day, Laura was proving to be a mature, highly self-directed student and successfully met the course objectives. In fact, the second preceptor did not observe any unprofessional behaviors.

While many aspects to this scenario are positive, the faculty regret the fact that the preceptor did not want to have anything to do with Laura after her removal. In the faculty's conference with Laura, the student posed the question of going to the preceptor and apologizing for her behavior. Instead she was advised to write a letter to the preceptor, outlining what had gone on. Under a different set of circumstances, the faculty believe the preceptor would have seen a very different student.

In situations where a student is clearly unsafe, the implementation of school policies and procedures related to unsafe performance should pose no problems in the precepted course. Due process is essential with all *evaluative* statements emanating from the faculty, not the preceptor.

Preceptor Role

Broadly speaking, the role of the preceptor is to bridge the gap between the reality of the workplace and the idealism of an academic environment without compromising professional ideals. Above all else, honest and open communication will establish a positive learning environment. The following responsibilities are germane to the preceptor. The preceptor should:

1. contract with the student for a specific period of time for the clinical experiences during the semester;
2. collaborate with the student to develop learning experiences congruent with the student's goals and objectives;
3. provide specific and effective ongoing feedback to the student through verbal and written communications;
4. communicate with faculty as to the student's progress and the nature of his or her overall learning experience; and
5. be open to the need to change and grow.

Unfortunately, many of these responsibilities cannot be substituted for, but are added to, the many patient and unit responsibilities of the preceptor. A workshop may be an effective means for helping preceptors identify strategies for balancing these multiple demands.

Student Role

The student's role in a precepted course is essentially the same as that typical of a traditional clinical course. With a full understanding of the course and clinical objectives, students will be formulating individualized learning objectives. Unlike the traditional method, the student will be sharing these objectives with an additional individual, the preceptor. One real strength of the precepted experience is the individualized attention the student can receive in formulating and revising learning objectives. Who has more knowledge of the rich learning opportunities available on the unit than the preceptor? The student's role is to tap this wealth of information. Situation 3-2 describes these advantages.

Situation 3-2

Learning Opportunities

For many years, faculty have supervised students in the traditional manner of bringing a group of 8–10 students onto a general medical-surgical unit and providing as many learning experiences as possible. Although faculty required each student to write individualized learning goals, their accomplishment was constrained by time (presence on the unit restricted to Thursdays and Fridays), patient availability (24 beds) and staffing patterns. To observe a cardiac catheterization was not an option, because it was only done on Mondays and Wednesdays. Most, if not all, students wrote psychomotor learning goals related to parenteral medications or sterile procedures. At the conclusion of the semester, it was not unusual for some of the students to have missed the opportunity for one or more of these experiences. A course utilizing preceptors changes all of that.

In the process of creating and piloting a required precepted course, faculty had no idea of the extent of learning opportunities that would become available to students. The logistics of the course required the student to spend 126 hours over seven weeks with a preceptor in a selected area of interest. These 126 hours average approximately 18 hours per week; however, faculty caution the students not to confine themselves in this manner. Rather, the objective is to show 126 hours of clinical time at the end of seven weeks (some weeks may be 24 hours, other weeks 8 hours). Students are expected to negotiate with the preceptors and fit the hours in around their other school class times. Consequently, students may spend an occasional weekend with the preceptor and, oftentimes, students are never in the clinical area on the same two days in successive weeks.

The flexibility in scheduling, coupled with the lack of competition for learning activities on the unit (usually only one or two students are precepted on any one unit) open a number of doors to the student. The cancer center, consisting of two medical units, a surgical unit, an ICU and an ambulatory clinic, was one of the first to become involved in the course and provide a wonderful example of that wealth of learning opportunities. When students were precepted on one of the oncology units, they were offered the following opportunities as part of their total clinical experience: observational days on the other units, as well as in surgery, observing one of the ongoing support groups, and participation in any of the core oncology courses offered to the staff. Because there are only one or two students on the unit, the entire staff becomes very vested in the students' learning, offering multiple opportunities to observe and practice complex procedures.

Once the door to learning has been opened, students, on the whole, become eager and creative in identifying other learning opportunities. For example, several of the students became involved in the data collection of a faculty member's ongoing coping study of cancer patients.

Self-Direction

While self-direction is a quality faculty look for and demand of all students, it is a must in a preceptorship. The advantage in a preceptorship is the support faculty can often gain from the preceptor in encouraging students to be self-directed. Often students are shocked when they find they are expected to devise their own clinical schedules. For some this first assignment is problematic. Students have available to them information regarding the flexibility of their clinical days and are advised that they may be expected to work weekends and off shifts with their preceptors. When given this information early, students are able and willing to make the necessary changes in their lives.

Accountability

Another aspect to self-direction is that of accountability. Prior to this precepted course students are held accountable by requiring preclinical preparation time, thereby giving them the time and opportunity to acquire the necessary knowledge and skills for safe practice. The precepted course usually is the first course where students cannot prepare ahead of time. It is the belief of faculty involved in the course that last semester seniors need to be exposed to situations where they have to effectively and efficiently obtain the essential information for safe practice in the work setting. Preparation must be defined differently in a preceptorship. The knowledge the student brings is not as important as the student's accountability in finding the answers. From the start, the faculty tell the student that the statement, "I don't know" must be followed with "but I will look it up before (giving the medication, doing the procedure)." Consequently, most students bring a number of required texts to their clinical sites.

Assertiveness

Assertiveness is another facet to self-direction that faculty need to require and nurture in the student. Often students are placed in somewhat passive roles in the traditional clinical setting. They are competing for limited learning opportunities, and a certain amount of luck determines whether or not the student will be selected for the particular learning opportunity. Since this competition is greatly reduced in preceptorships, students must articulate their learning needs to their preceptors each time they are with them. Experienced preceptors are often quite adept in helping students identify and accomplish selected learning goals. Students working with new preceptors may need some guidance in reminding the preceptor what it is they want from the experience.

THE SELECTION PROCESS

For all three members of the preceptorship relationship, a process of selecting individuals for a precepted course should be considered. The following discussion highlights some of the more important issues to consider.

Selecting the Faculty

Length of teaching experience and the ability to delegate student supervision are the two most important criteria in selecting faculty to teach a precepted course. Generally speaking, faculty lacking these attributes are not well suited to manage a precepted course. Direct supervision is largely delegated to the preceptor. Related activities, such as asking students about their preparation, identifying appropriate patient assignments, and observing student-patient interactions, are no longer part of the faculty role.

Selecting the Preceptor

Considerable control can be exercised when selecting preceptors. In deciding whether someone should be a preceptor, the foremost issue is their willingness to be a preceptor, particularly in light of the declining resources available for rewarding such behavior. The second consideration is credentials and, finally, the length of the nurse's experience. No preceptor who has fewer than 18 months experience should be used. Many state boards for nursing education stipulate that preceptors must possess the minimum of a bachelor-of-science degree in nursing in order to precept an undergraduate baccalaureate student. Another credential to consider is certification in one's subspecialty, such as oncology (Oncology Nursing Society). Such credentialing indicates a commitment to professional development.

There are other factors to consider in the selection process, which are italicized in the following paragraphs.

When considering the nurse's *length of experience in the particular specialty*, explore where the experience has been. For example, a nurse with five years medical-surgical experience, but who is new (less than one year) to the field of neuroscience, may not be the best candidate for a neuroscience preceptorship.

Seek a *recommendation from the preceptor's immediate supervisor*. Data regarding the preceptor's professional practice, judgement, and decision-making skills, communication skills, clinical expertise, mentoring skills and enthusiasm for the role should be assessed by the supervisor.

Assess whether the nurse's *work schedule will fit with the student's school schedule*. While a number of part-time staff display many of the attributes of a good preceptor, unless they work at least 30 hours a week, the student will have difficulty acquiring the necessary time to achieve the course objectives. A variation on this is the weekend-alternative staff. Given the increasing diversity of students, weekend-alternative clinical experience may be very appealing to students with small children who can better fit into this schedule. The disadvantage is the student's lack of exposure to the regular work-week environment of the agency.

Student Selection

Students cannot be selected for a precepted course based on credentials or other attributes, particularly if it is a required course. Rather than a selection process, students undergo an education or orientation process to the role of preceptee. As a preceptee, the student will often be the only student on the unit, and finding immediate support from peers may not be easy. Where there is considerable latitude in placing students, student input regarding placement may help alleviate the sense of isolation often felt while on the unit.

DESIGNING AND IMPLEMENTING A PRECEPTED COURSE

With a full understanding of the roles and responsibilities of the faculty, student, and preceptor, faculty should find designing a precepted course similar to designing a traditional clinical course. In fact, any clinical course can utilize preceptors. Much depends on the role which faculty wish the preceptors to play in the course. The course described here requires the student to synthesize previously learned material and to develop a personal philosophy of nursing. A preceptorship plays a critical role in helping the student meet these requirements.

Placement in the Curriculum

The Senior Clinical Practicum is the student's final clinical course before graduation with all courses in the program being either pre- or co-requisites to the practicum. The course is described in extremely broad terms, thus allowing student placements in a variety of settings. Students are encouraged to identify their own placements and have shown considerable creativity in doing so. Since its inception in 1992, the Senior Clinical Practicum has facilitated the placement of students in such diverse settings as ambulatory clinics, school-based clinics, rehabilitation facilities, extended-care facilities, and the usual acute-care settings. The only restriction in placement is that requests for placement with Advance Practice Nurses (midwives, nurse anesthetists, nurse practitioners) are not considered appropriate.

POLICIES AND PROCEDURES

Even the most self-directed, mature student needs some structure. In designing the precepted course, faculty have found that having some policies and procedures will help provide that structure. There have been mixed reviews (from faculty and preceptors) on the policies, most notable is the rigidity of the policies. Students, on the other hand, have found them workable. Tables 3-1 and 3-2 list the policies, procedures, and scheduling guidelines, respectively, for a precepted course.

TABLE 3-1   Clinical Policies and Procedures

The following *student* responsibilities have been found to be important:

---

1. Students must participate in a clinical unit orientation.
2. A clinical schedule must be submitted to the faculty with each new work schedule. Faculty must approve clinical schedules. All changes in clinical schedules must be approved by faculty. Hours not approved are subject to "make up" time. Failure to submit student schedules, changes or logs result in deficiencies on the Clinical Evaluation Tool (CET).
3. Student's scheduling night clinical experience must verify safe transportation to and from the hospital. UNIVERSITY POLICE ESCORTS ARE AVAILABLE—USE GOOD JUDGEMENT!
4. Students are expected to arrive at least fifteen minutes before the start of clinical experience.
5. Students who are reporting absent need to call the unit, speak to the nurse in charge, leave a message for the *pre-*

*ceptor, and not*ify faculty at least one hour prior to clinical experience.

6. Students should be assigned to only the preceptor's patients. Since the preceptor is ultimately responsible for the care administered to patients, regular assessment and follow-up of student care is to be expected.

7. Primary care is only to be provided to the assigned patient. However, supervised therapies or observations of other patients on the units can occur at the discretion of the preceptor.

8. Any student signature needs to be co-signed by the preceptor. This is to be validated as part of the end-of-shift routine.

9. Students should be supervised for all invasive procedures (e.g., catheterizations, suctioning, etc.) by the preceptor.

10. All incident reports involving the student or student's clients need to be co-signed by the preceptor, and faculty must be notified.

11. Students must be supervised for ALL MEDICATIONS administered.

12. Students are *required* to attend weekly seminars with faculty. Times to be announced.

13. All written assignments must be submitted to faculty on time (as specified by faculty)! Faculty will grade assignments and return them to students in the clinical area.

14. Midterm and final clinical evaluations will be conducted formally by the faculty. Students are responsible for self-evaluations at this time.

15. Students obtaining deficiencies during the rotation must meet with faculty to outline areas for improvement and plan to meet each clinical day to review and document progress.

16. Students need to take responsibility for learning, and must seek guidance as appropriate.

17. ILLNESS OR INJURY: Students can be referred to student health (or appropriate service). If such service is lacking on

continued

TABLE 3-1   *continued*

evening and nights, students should be referred to the
emergency room. Faculty should be notified as soon as
possible.

18. PRECEPTOR IS ILL: Another preceptor may be able to fol-
    low the student. An alternative experience can also be
    arranged if necessary. For example, an ICU observation or
    Ambulatory Care observation might be an appropriate
    alternative.

19. INCIDENT REPORTS: The faculty should be notified as
    soon as possible that an incident has occurred. The precep-
    tor should co-sign the report and faculty will follow-up.

20. WHEN STUDENT IS NOT PREPARED OR NEEDS REME-
    DIATION: Faculty will assist these students, but should be
    notified as soon as possible so that the student can be
    removed from the unit and taken to skills labs, counseling,
    etc.

21. STUDENT ABSENCE: Students are required to notify fac-
    ulty of illness or inability to attend clinical. This time must
    be made up under the supervision of the preceptor or an
    approved substitute.

22. SCHEDULE CHANGES: Students are required to get
    approval from the faculty prior to schedule changes.

23. SAFETY AND HONESTY: Students are to refer to the aca-
    demic institution's student handbook regarding the poli-
    cies on "Unsafe Clinical Performance of Nursing Students"
    and "Academic Dishonesty"

Grading Policies

As stated earlier, clinical objectives are Pass/Fail and all objectives
are derived from earlier courses. Clinical objectives must be attain-
able in all settings and therefore, are stated in very broad terms.
The student is evaluated in the following areas:

1. Professional behavior;
2. Nurse-client relationship;

3. The Nursing Process: Assessment, Analysis, Planning, Implementation, and Evaluation; and
4. Assimilation as a Member of the Health Team.

In addition to the clinical component, there is a weekly, two-hour seminar that provides the didactic component of the course. Students are graded on their seminar participation, documentation of clinical logs, and a clinical leadership project.

The clinical leadership project, worth 45 percent of the grade, is the faculty's technique for bridging clinical experience and theory. Students are expected to identify, design, and implement a patient- or staff-centered teaching project. Collaboration with their preceptors and other staff members in identifying a relevant topic is an essential component of the requirement. The project is also the faculty's way of thanking the staff for their efforts in the student's education. As part of their grade, students submit a five-page paper describing the process of assessing the unit's needs, rationale for topic selection, and the actual product (e.g., poster, pamphlet, handouts, booklets). Feedback from preceptors is sought as to the appropriateness and adequacy of the project.

Student case presentations in the seminars are utilized to explore the following course objectives:

1. Identify researchable questions in a selected clinical area;
2. Demonstrate leadership abilities in the proactive, reactive, and collaborative provision of nursing care in a selected clinical area;
3. Demonstrate the integration of the empirical, ethical, personal, and aesthetic perspectives in professional decision-making and practice;
4. Analyze the interrelationships of the environmental contexts and human responses unique to a selected clinical area; and
5. Evaluate the impact of cost, access, and quality of care in relation to selected client populations.

Clinical Sites

In the semester prior to the course's first time offering, letters are sent to every clinical facility that has an affiliation with the school.

In the letter, the course, the roles of faculty, student, and preceptor are described. Facilities are asked about their potential interest in having students in this capacity. This approach will identify agencies unable to participate because of internal policies (e.g., faculty must be on-site, no unlicensed precepted students) and staffing restrictions.

During pre-registration for the course, a "Clinical Preference Questionnaire" is distributed to students. The form asks: (1) for the student's ranking of a number of clinical specialties (adult health, community health, pediatrics) and sub-specialties (oncology, neuroscience, neonatal); (2) if there is a particular agency of interest; (3) their use of transportation; and (4) in what geographical part of the state they wish to be placed. Students are then placed with consideration given to their preferences, whenever possible.

As the course has matured, students have been given an increasing amount of freedom to find their own clinical facility. Table 3-2 describes the process for a student initiated clinical placement.

TABLE 3-2   Policies and Procedures for Student Initiated Clinicals

1. Students may not be precepted by a family member or personal acquaintance.

2. In general, students may not be precepted on a unit where they are currently employed. In rare circumstances, with full cooperation and understanding from the nurse manager, a student may be precepted on the unit, but it must be on a shift that the student normally does not work.

3. To be a preceptor, a staff nurse must have a minimum of a baccalaureate in nursing and have at least 18 months experience.

4. If a student has a particular preceptor in mind, he or she is to forward to the course coordinator, *in writing*, at least one month prior to the first day of class, the following:

   a) name of preceptor, credentials, and years of experience;

   b) clinical facility, type of unit, and unit phone number;

   c) name and phone of preceptor's first-line supervisor
      (usually this is the nurse manager);

     d) name and phone number of the director of staff development, or the equivalent person in charge of student placements in the particular unit.

5. If a student has a particular clinical facility in mind, he or she is to forward to the course coordinator, *in writing*, at least one month prior to the first day of class, the following:

     a) name and phone number of the clinical facility and director of staff development or the equivalent person in charge of student placements in the facility.

Some facilities, particularly those utilized by a number of different nursing programs, have requested only faculty contact for student placements. Smaller, less frequently utilized facilities have embraced the notion of working with students to find a suitable placement. By giving students this freedom there is less pressure on faculty to contact so many facilities. Faculty have also found students who establish their own sites to be more enthusiastic about the experience.

Some issues regarding clinical placements have surfaced. The most prevalent and reoccurring are the appropriateness of the intensive care units for student placements and the impact of health care reform on availability of acute-care sites.

The Intensive Care Unit as an Appropriate Site for Students: Yes or No?

Far more students request the Intensive Care Unit (ICU) than there are available placements. Because this is a required course and faculty believe all students should have equal opportunity for their priority placements, a lottery system is utilized to select students.

The more compelling issue for faculty and ICU nurse managers is the role of the ICU in a clinical course. Prior to this course most student experiences in the ICU have been observational. That is not the case in the Senior Clinical Practicum. Over the years, faculty have found student experiences to be much more positive in those settings where Nurse Managers hire new graduates. Staff in these settings are expert in identifying and addressing the anxieties and limited skills of the novice nurse. A similar expertise is not consistently found in ICUs that routinely do not hire new graduates. Consequently, at this time, at our facility we try to avoid placement of students in such settings.

With increasing numbers of hospital beds closing, competition is becoming ever more fierce for nursing student placements in acute-care settings. By the same token, while the numbers of patients receiving nursing care in the home and in ambulatory settings has increased, equivalent numbers of appropriate student placements have not occurred. Finally, enrollment in nursing schools remains at an all time high. Consequently, faculty and students have had to become ever more creative in identifying appropriate practicum sites. As a nursing school located within an academic health center, our primary facilities have been university-based teaching hospitals. With increased student involvement, faculty have had extremely positive experiences with small community-based and rural hospitals.

A PRECEPTOR WORKSHOP

While the components to a preceptor workshop are presented as the last section to this chapter, this does not mean to imply a lack of importance. The faculty have discovered a world of difference in those preceptors who attend the workshop and those who are oriented to the course on an individual basis. In addition to all participants hearing the same information in the workshop, the setting provides multiple opportunities for preceptors to exchange ideas, process information more slowly and completely, and to voice well thought out questions.

Workshop Topics

The workshop is one-half day, continuing education units are awarded, and the following topics are explored:

1. Curriculum overview and course description;
2. Roles: Faculty, student, preceptor;

3. Teaching strategies and the adult learner;
4. Describing student performance versus evaluating student performance; and
5. Legal ramifications to precepting unlicensed students.

Curriculum Overview and Course Description

Participants are introduced to the school's curriculum and are shown how the student arrives at the senior practicum. Preceptors are given a course description, which includes course objectives, course requirements, and ways in which students will be evaluated. Policies and procedures for the course are also reviewed (see Table 3-1).

Roles: Faculty, Student, Preceptor

Participants are given essentially the same information on roles that was presented earlier in this chapter. As the various roles are discussed and explored, participants who have precepted licensed individuals usually have a number of questions related to role delineation. Such areas as how to use the faculty and under what circumstances does one hold (or not hold) the student accountable are the most frequently asked questions.

Teaching Strategies and the Adult Learner

While all nurses are educated to and have assumed the role of teacher, the participants' perspective is often narrowly limited to patients. The goal of the preceptor workshop is to broaden that perspective by having a guest speaker review case scenarios and by asking participants to reflect on their own educational experiences.

The guest speaker cautions participants to be aware of a number of phenomena that can greatly affect the teaching-learning environment. In addition to the obvious ones of patient emotional responses, presence of other health care providers, and changes in patient status, the participants also learn and are encouraged to include strategies such as role-playing and problem-solving using case studies. Other important topics include conflict resolution, role-modeling, and effective ways to motivate students.

Describing Student Performance versus Evaluating Student Performance

Although the roles of the preceptor and faculty are delineated early in the workshop, special consideration is given to a more thorough exploration of student evaluations. Participants express confusion and anxiety with regard to this process. A number of clinical examples are used to reinforce their role. Of greater anxiety to the faculty are those preceptors who are unable to tell students their weaknesses and yet express to the faculty serious reservations regarding the student's abilities to be safe.

Due process is an important theme during the presentation of this topic. The need to keep both student and faculty apprised of student performance is emphasized. The relationship between student performance and achieving clinical objectives is also emphasized.

Because it is not possible for all staff nurses to attend the workshop, a manual that summarizes the workshop's essential information has been developed. This manual is used when orienting any new preceptors who are unable to attend the workshop. Preceptors who have used the manual have found it useful and have been determined to be equally prepared as those attending the workshop.

Legal Ramifications to Precepting Unlicensed Students

The guest speaker for this topic is a nurse educator who is also a lawyer. Using the state's Nurse Practice Act as the overriding framework, the guest speaker reviews the concepts of negligence, malpractice, and legal accountability as they relate to the Nurse Practice Act and precepting. Several legal cases involving student nurses are utilized as the basis for exploring the legal duties and responsibilities of the student, preceptor, and faculty. This topic generates a number of questions from the audience and has been consistently highly rated in the workshop evaluations.

SUMMARY

This chapter has presented the process of developing and implementing an undergraduate preceptorship. The roles and responsibilities of the student, preceptor, and faculty were explored and linked to the success of an undergraduate preceptorship. The importance of maintaining clear, open lines of communication was a theme throughout the chapter. A number of factors related to selecting appropriate preceptors and faculty were described. A model undergraduate preceptorship was used to highlight important policies and procedures. Finally, a workshop preparing staff nurses for the preceptor role was described.

REFERENCES

Chickerella, B. G., & Lutz, W. J. (1981). Professional nurturance: Preceptorships for undergraduate nursing students. *American Journal of Nursing, 81,* 107–109.

Donius, M. A. H. (1988). The Columbia precepting program: Building a bridge with clinical faculty. *Journal of Professional Nursing, 4,* 17–22.

Goldenberg, D. (1987/1988). Preceptorship: A one-to-one relationship with a triple "P" rating (preceptor, preceptee, patient). *Nursing Forum, 23(1),* 10–15.

Hseih, N. L., & Knowles, D. W. (1990). Instructor facilitation of the preceptorship relationship in nursing education. *Journal of Nursing Education, 29(6),* 262–268.

Scales, F. S., Alverson, E. & Harder, D. L. (1993). The effect of a preceptorship on nursing performance. *Nursing Connections, 6(2),* 45–54.

Scheetz, L. J. (1989). Baccalaureate nursing student preceptorship programs and the development of clinical competence. *Journal of Nursing Education, 28(1),* 29–35.

SUGGESTED READINGS

Konkel, J., Soares, P., & Russler, M. (1994). A collaborative framework for baccalaureate clinical preceptorships. *Journal of Nursing Staff Development, 10(2)*, 94-98.

McKnight, J., Black, M., Latta, E., & Parsons, M. (1993). Preceptor workshops: A collaborative model. *Nursing Connections, 6(3)*, 5–14.

Reilly, D. E., & Oerman, M. H. (1992). *Clinical teaching in nursing education*. New York: National League for Nursing.

Zerbe, M. A., & Lachat, M. F. (1991). A three-tiered team model for undergraduate preceptor programs. *Nurse Educator, 16(2)*, 18–21.

Chapter **4**

AN ON-THE-JOB PRECEPTOR MODEL FOR NEWLY HIRED NURSES

Janet Mackin, RNC, MS, CNA
Kathleen Studva, RN, MA

T his chapter focuses on a preceptorship for nurse orientees in major health care organizations. The assumption is that the preceptorship is designed by a nurse educator who assumes responsibility for the program and for negotiating among orientees, preceptor, and nurser manager. While the chapter is specific to this situation, many of the principles and practices discussed here would apply to other preceptorships as well.

This chapter provides preparatory information to:

- design a preceptor training program; and
- implement the preceptor role in the clinical setting.

DESIGNING A PRECEPTOR PROGRAM

Before getting into the specifics of designing a preceptor program, it is important to take an overview of the health-care facility, the philosophy of the nursing department, the clinical and educational competence of the nursing staff, and the educational philosophy of the department. The goal is to develop a preceptor program that is well integrated within the structure of the health-care facility. An initial overall assessment will prevent adoption of a cookie-cutter model for a preceptor program, making the work a little more difficult but far more worthwhile.

As a starter, ask the following questions:

- **"What are the current mission, strategic plan, and specific goals of the health-care facility?** Not only should the mission and goals of the institution be implicitly and explicitly included in the content of the preceptor program, but it should also be used as a guide to the program's design as well. In the rapidly changing health-care field, the mission of an institution can change dramatically. For example, an institutional switch from an emphasis on in-patient services to out-patient services would change the mission and should also be reflected in the design of the preceptor program. Or, if improving patient satisfaction is high on the institution's list of goals, a customer relations component should be included in the functions of the preceptors and orientees. Case studies, orientee evaluation tools, and specific content may need to be adjusted to reflect these types of institutional changes.

- **"What are the philosophy, conceptual framework, and mission of the Nursing Department in the institution?"** The answer to this question should be consistent with the institutional mission and goals, but it should also provide some additional insights that will be important to one's preceptor program. For example, preceptors should be more than familiar with the philosophy of the nursing department; they should be able to explain, apply, and, if necessary, defend it. This does not mean that they need to memorize the philosophy, but that they should feel its impact and implications in their practice. In addition, if one's nursing department utilizes a specific conceptual framework, the preceptor program should be reviewed for consistency with each component of the framework.

- **"What is the level of the nursing staff's clinical competence?"** In some institutions, one has the luxury of working with a highly skilled, experienced nursing staff. Under these

circumstances, preceptor selection will not present a problem and the development of the learners' educational skills
will be easier. The preceptor program for this group can be
of a high caliber and comprehensive. On the other hand, the
staff may be a group of fledglings in a new area of practice,
who are having a difficult time finding their own way.
Selecting the most prepared of these nurses for preceptor
training may require an evaluation of the nurse's potential
for precepting rather than demonstrated performance. More
often, however, one selects preceptors from a mixed group
of practitioners. In designing a preceptor program for a
diverse group, the match between learner and preceptor is
important. One wants to build-in an opportunity for the
more savvy preceptors to share their insights and experience
with those learners who are a little shaky about a new role.
Pre-program preparatory activities may help put preceptors
and learners at more equal starting points.

- **"What is the educational philosophy of the nursing education department?"** The most likely answer to this question
  is "an adult education philosophy." The principles of
  Malcolm Knowles have become a standard feature in nursing education. If these principles were swallowed whole,
  however, one may find inconsistencies between what is said
  and what is done. For example, to say that learners are self-
  directed, yet control their educational activities sets a bad
  educational model. It might be more honest and accurate to
  acknowledge the fact that, in an institutional setting, minimum educational standards are set by the institution and
  that learners need to be guided to meet these requirements.
  Nor should one overlook the fact that adults need to learn at
  their own speed. What are the options for a slow learner
  remediating or an experienced nurse opting out of the program? If the program designer does not challenge herself on
  her ability to practice what she preaches, her preceptors will.

Taking the time to think through the implications of answers to
the above questions will help to situate the preceptor program
appropriately in the institution. A generic approach to designing a
preceptor program will fail to meet the needs of the preceptors,
orientees, and the institution.

Criteria for Preceptor Selection

As part of the design of the preceptor training program, prerequisites for preceptor selection should be developed and then shared with the nurse managers. The nurse manager will need to be involved in identifying staff members eligible for the training program. Some suggested prerequisites include the following:

- An ability to role model professional behavior;
- demonstrated support of the philosophy of the nursing department;
- an ability to communicate effectively; and
- a desire to precept new staff members.

You will need to define the specific criteria for each of the prerequisites. For example, you may define each of the prerequisites in a fashion similar to those shown in Table 4-1.

TABLE 4-1   Criteria for Preceptor Selection

An ability to role model professional practice

1. Successful completion of all aspects of orientation to the assigned unit.
2. Performance evaluation that exceeds the minimum requirements.
3. Current proficiency in all items identified on the unit-specific skills monitor.
4. Current Basic Cardiac Life Support/Advanced Cardiac Life Support certification.
5. Mandatory educational requirements fulfilled.

Demonstrated support of the philosophy of the nursing department

6. Participation in at least one nursing committee, a hospital committee, or a unit-based project.
7. Willingness to assume charge responsibilities as necessary.

An ability to communicate effectively

8. Gives accurate, efficient, and effective shift reports.
9. Delivers clear, appropriate, and accurate patient education.
10. Communicates well with all members of the interdisciplinary team.

A Desire to Precept New Staff Members

11. Has completed application/assessment form for Preceptor Training Program.
12. Has conducted informal staff education activities.

During the Preceptor Training Program, the selection criteria should be reviewed with the preceptor candidates. This initial feedback will help reinforce the preceptor's commitment to the program and the new role. The preceptors are made to feel special from the program's onset.

Characteristics of the Adult Learner

It is important to include a review of adult learner characteristics (see Chapter 2) as part of the core content of the preceptor program. Frequently, the preceptors have been exposed to adult education concepts and principles during their basic education and, hopefully, during their orientation to the institution. However, at these times the preceptors were on the receiving end of the educational process and were focusing on the educational content, rather than the educational strategies. As preceptors, they will need to utilize adult education strategies to enable the orientee to succeed. The ability to understand the adult learner will greatly assist in orientee assessment and appropriate assignment planning.

Roles and Responsibilities

There are usually four professionals involved in the orientation process: the orientee, the preceptor, the nurse manager, and the nurse educator. Everyone should be clear regarding his/her individual responsibilities. During the preceptor program, an outline of the specific responsibilities assigned to each role should be reviewed in order to provide the preceptor with a clear description of expected roles. The following are examples of responsibilities that might be assigned to each of the roles.

Orientee Responsibilities

- With the assistance of the preceptor and the nurse educator, identifies goals and objectives for orientation based on learning needs.
- Utilizes available resources to meet learning needs.
- Assumes increasing responsibility for patient care with preceptor guidance.
- Participates with the preceptor, nurse manager, and nurse educator in the appraisal process.
- Evaluates the orientation program including the preceptor component.

Preceptor Responsibilities

- Attends the Preceptor Training Program.
- With the orientee and nurse educator, identifies goals and objectives for orientation based upon learning needs.
- Serves as a bridge for the orientee's social integration into the unit.
- Plans orientee's assignment, based upon the orientee's input and an objective assessment.
- Role models professional practice for the orientee.
- Acts as a clinical resource and support.
- Provides feedback to the orientee, the nurse manager, and the nurse educator.
- Identifies problems and refers them to the nurse manager and the nurse educator.
- Coordinates the orientee's clinical assignment with the orientation content.
- Utilizes orientation tools.

- Participates in the appraisal process with the orientee, the nurse manager, and the nurse educator.
- Evaluates the Preceptor Program.

Nurse Manager Responsibilities

- Selects a preceptor for each orientee.
- Schedules preceptor's time and assignment to ensure availability for the orientee.
- Supports the preceptor and the orientee in problem identification.
- Provides feedback to the preceptor and the orientee.
- Participates in the appraisal process with the orientee, the preceptor, and the nurse educator.
- Evaluates the Preceptor Program.

Nurse Educator Responsibilities

- Provides the orientee with general orientation content.
- Assists the nurse manager in selecting a preceptor for each orientee.
- Assists the preceptor and the orientee in identifying the goals and objectives for the orientation, based upon learning needs.
- Role models professional practice for the preceptor.
- Provides preceptor training, guidance, support, and feedback.
- Assists the preceptor and the orientee in problem identification and provides additional instruction or clinical supervision when indicated.
- Participates in the appraisal process with the orientee, the preceptor, and the nurse manager.
- Evaluates the preceptor.

Orientee Assessment and Socialization

To enable the orientee to move through the system and assume the responsibilities of a full working staff member, the preceptor has to be able to assess the orientees' skills and progress, as well as to socialize the orientee to the working environment. During an initial assessment, the preceptor will need to ascertain the following:

- The orientee's educational background and past work experience;
- The orientee's self-assessment data; and
- The orientee's self-report of concerns or fears.

To do an ongoing assessment of the orientee's abilities, the preceptor will need to provide a variety of meaningful clinical experiences and advance appropriately their difficulty and level of responsibility. The preceptor's hesitation to advance the level of assignments of an orientee beyond that of an assistant needs to be challenged. An important role of the preceptor is to observe the orientee's performance and question them for further clarification of their clinical activities. During the program the preceptor should learn to appreciate the fact that assessment skills correlate closely with adult education concepts. The more preceptors understand their assessment responsibilities as they relate to the adult learner, the clearer will become the concept that orientation or learning is a shared responsibility.

The preceptor not only serves as an "on the spot resource" for clinical situations, but also facilitates the orientee's integration into the unit's social milieu. Ways to accomplish this should be covered in the Preceptor Training Program. The following are presented as simple suggestions:

- Introduce the orientee to unit personnel and other members of the health care team.
- Review the unit's system for patient care delivery.
- Provide information regarding roles and responsibilities of the members of the health care team.
- Involve the orientee in unit activities and routines.

Learning Styles

The Preceptor Training Program is an excellent opportunity to familiarize clinical experts with the concept of learning styles. Typically the clinical experts expect all learners to assimilate information in a fashion similar to their own. The rationale goes thus:"I learned to become a good nurse by *(observing others/studying the theory/practicing/experimenting/etc.).* . . . and it worked for me. Therefore, it is the best way to learn for every new nurse." The logic derived from personal experience can be misleading and often inhibits the preceptor's ability to understand the learning styles of others.

At a minimum, the Preceptor Training Program should include a review of the basic learning styles. Either the work of Kolb (1993), Gregorc (1984), or Honey and Mumford (1989) can be selected as a model for understanding learning styles. Unfortunately, if presented as pure theory, the import and impact of this information may not be appreciated by the preceptors. A more experiential model for teaching learning styles may be more effective. The following exercise (Mulqueen, 1995) is an example of a participative method for presenting teaching learning styles. In this example, the Kolb Learning Style Inventory is used, but other learning assessment tools can be used in a similar fashion.

Exercise 1. Learning Styles

At the beginning of the program, all preceptors complete a learning style assessment. Scored assessments reveal each individual's learning style. At a later point in the program, participants are grouped at tables according to their learning styles. There is no need to tell the participants why they are assigned to a particular group. Most frequently, there is a rather equal distribution of learning styles within a class. The group assignment is to create an object that represents the group. Colored paper, markers, old magazines, and any other interesting objects may be used by the group.

Educators who have done this exercise over and over again are amazed at the consistency of the results. If the Kolb Learning Styles Inventory is used, for example, the groups that prefer "Active Experimentation" and "Concrete Experience" are usually complaining that there are not enough supplies. They use up every minute feverishly building their object. The people whose learning styles fall into the categories of "Abstract Conceptualization" and "Reflective Observation" are usually slow to execute the project. These type of learners frequently need to clarify the rules and the purpose of the exercise and are somewhat embarrassed about their lack of activity. However, their thoughtful probing of the issue usually reveals some surprising insights.

At the end of the exercise time is allocated to review each of the learning styles, allowing members from each of the groups to give examples of the group's learning style. For example, members of the "Abstract Conceptualization" group are likely to bring up the fact they needed to have a theory of what their object would be before they could start construction. "Concrete Experience" group members may state that they felt better once they got their hands on the materials they would be using.

The facilitator of this session will need to lead the groups in further discussion of how this information can be used when they are precepting an orientee. Having discovered their own learning style preference and seeing that it is not the only way of learning, preceptors are more likely to be tolerant of orientees whose learning styles are different from their own. In addition, by providing a learning activity that allows for concrete experience, active experimentation, abstract conceptualization, as well as reflective observation, the Preceptor Training Program facilitator is able to model and reinforce the information regarding learning styles (Mulqueen, 1995).

Cultural Diversity

Preceptor candidates are usually familiar with some aspects of cultural diversity. Basic nursing school curricula usually include a component dealing with issues of cultural diversity as they pertain to patients. However, including information on cultural diversity in a preceptor program is also recommended. With the influx of large numbers of foreign nurses and the mobility of nurses within the United States, the probability is high that a preceptor will be asked to work with an orientee from a substantially different cultural, religious, or ethnic background. During the Preceptor

Training Program, the topic of cultural diversity should be examined from a variety of viewpoints. Consider including some of the following approaches:

Cultural Stereotypes and How They Influence Our Expectations. Even those most critically aware of how cultural stereotyping influences behavior need a "booster shot" from time to time. For those less aware of their hidden assumptions regarding cultural differences, program content on diversity is an opportunity for them to explore their thoughts and feelings on the topic. For those with blatant prejudices, a cultural diversity program is essential to either change their opinions or to prevent them from inflicting their prejudices on orientees. Consider using prepackaged, professionally produced programs or developing an exercise activity. One effective class exercise is to form teams and have participants identify as many commonly held stereotypes as possible for different cultural groups. For example, one group would be assigned to list stereotypes associated with HispanicAmericans, another group would do the same for AfricanAmericans, another group for AsianAmericans. On completing the lists, the class as a whole could analyze how many of the stereotypes are negative. The group could also be prompted to examine how quickly and easily they were able to make the lists which indicates how prevalent these prejudices are in society. Utilizing educators who are sensitive to cultural diversity issues is important to the success of this exercise. A team-teaching approach can work very well, especially if the team is culturally diverse.

Cultural Transition Processes and Issues Preceptors need to have an awareness of some of the physical, emotional, educational, and social transitions required of foreign or newly relocated staff members. Although these nurses most likely have a theoretical awareness of the difficulty of making a transition, they may need assistance in gaining a sensitivity and true appreciation for just how difficult these transitions can be. Storytelling can be an excellent method for approaching these issues in the affective domain. Allowing preceptors to share their own experiences of transition with the group is one way in which participants can develop an empathy for the nurse experiencing a cultural transition.

Cultural Differences Related to Learning Styles and Professional Practice. There are specific facts about the education and professional practice of nurses from different cultures that need to be shared with preceptors. For example, nurses from the Philippines have a baccalaureate degree as their basic entry into practice, and in their country they are assisted in the personal care of their patients by a variety of the patient's family members and friends. With this information, preceptors will be able to help Filipino nurses deal with the different support systems and responsibilities nurses have in the United States. The presence or lack of a college degree in Nursing is important in the United States. Nurses from the Caribbean need to be prepared for this, since diploma schools still flourish in these countries. Nurses from Germany are accustomed to giving morning care at 3 or 4 A.M. and need to know that is not the practice in the United States. The list could go on and on. To present pertinent information of this nature to the preceptor group, consider using staff members from a variety of cultural backgrounds to give an overview on different nursing education and practice issues. An interview type session where the cultural representatives are interviewed by the preceptor group can be effective.

Problem-Solving Strategies. Whatever the time limitations of the Preceptor Training Program, it will be impossible to discuss all cultural diversity issues. Some time must be saved for discussing problem-solving strategies. The preceptor group should be encouraged to identify as many problem-solving techniques as possible. Their lists should include suggestions such as the following:

- Acting as orientee advocate;
- Assessing cultural issues routinely for all orientees;
- Validating behavior and clarifying expectations;
- Role-modeling; and
- Using culturally compatible preceptors.

Providing Feedback

Knowing how to provide feedback in a helpful, nonthreatening fashion is one of the most important qualities of a successful preceptor. This ability enhances the orientee's trust of the preceptor and the ability to hear what the preceptor is saying. During the

Preceptor Training Program, techniques for providing constructive feedback should be reviewed and practiced. Table 4-2 identifies some characteristics of helpful, nonthreatening feedback.

TABLE 4-2   Characteristics of Positive Feedback

- *Focusing on the behaviors rather than the inferences.* For example, "You finished all parts of the admission assessment except that the blood pressure was not recorded" is preferable to "Don't you know enough to take a patient's blood pressure when you admit them?"

- *Using descriptive rather than judgmental terms.* For example, "Your hand was shaking when you gave the injection" is preferable to "You were a nervous wreck."

- *Discussing specific situations rather than abstractions.* For example, "You seem to have had difficulty teaching Mrs. about her diabetic diet" is preferable to saying "You really have problems with patient teaching."

- *Sharing ideas rather than giving advice.* "Have you considered . . . " is a good opener for sharing ideas. In contrast "Listen to me . . . " narrows communication to a one-way street.

- *Exploring alternatives rather than providing solutions.* Asking questions, such as, "Can you think of any other way that you might handle the situation?" can yield interesting results, while a statement, such as, "There's only one thing you can do about it now" closes the door to creative thinking on the part of the orientee.

- *Limiting the amount of feedback at any one time.* Even the most motivated orientee is limited in the amount of feedback that can be processed at one time. Giving too much, too soon is like asking the orientee to drink from a fire hose rather than a fountain of wisdom.

- *Making sure that feedback is given in a respectful, confidential manner.* The center of the nurse's station is not a good location for giving feedback. Finding a quiet spot to discuss the orientee's progress demonstrates a caring, respectful concern for the new staff member.

- *Remembering that feedback is not a venting session for the preceptor.* Even the best preceptors can become frustrated with their orientees, and new preceptors need to be prepared to expect this. Preceptors need to identify venting techniques and support systems for themselves; otherwise, preceptors can inappropriately lash into an orientee, which results in *two* very embarrassed nurses.

Clinical Teaching

At the onset of the Preceptor Training Program, preceptors are reminded that they have been selected for the program because of their clinical expertise and their ability to role-model professional behavior. This is done as an acknowledgment of their achievement and as an enhancement for their self-esteem. As the program progresses, care must be taken to define clinical expertise more specifically, otherwise competent nurses can be intimidated by this notion of being "an expert." Making a step-by-step analysis of their abilities, preceptors can see their strengths and can identify their weaknesses as a part of their development as a nurse. In other words, preceptors need to acknowledge the fact that they are expert nurses but an expert nurse need not be a perfect nurse.

To conduct this step-by-step assessment, one reviews with preceptors the skills-assessment tools that are used in your institution. The purpose of making this assessment is twofold: it reinforces the competence and ability of the preceptors, and it will remind them of all the clinical skills that they will be assessing in the orientee. Preceptors should be able to perform all the skills on the assessment list. If, by chance, there are any skills that preceptors are lacking, this is an opportunity to direct preceptors on how they can update their skills.

Skills expected of a preceptor include:

- patient-care skills;
- organizational skills;
- problem-solving skills; and
- interpersonal skills with patients and co-workers.

The preceptor needs to be aware of the topics the orientee is reviewing in the orientation program, in order to plan assignments properly. For example, the preceptor needs to know that an orientee has completed the learning activities on medication administration before assigning medication responsibilities. During the clinical portion of orientation, the preceptor needs to provide progressive, challenging assignments that increase the orientee's independence. The preceptor must allow the orientee to "get his hands wet," but must also be ready to rescue the orientee who is drowning. Finally, the preceptor needs to document the clinical experiences with which the orientee has either assisted or has observed.

Orientation Model and Tools

Orientation calendars, schedules, assessment tools, guidelines, exercises, and resource materials are components of the orientation program with which preceptors should be familiar. Although preceptors were exposed to these materials as a part of their own orientation, the focus for them at that time was their own performance outcomes, not the tools. During the Preceptor Training Program, the purpose and use of each orientation tool needs to be spelled out in detail and the implications for the preceptor spelled out. Preceptors know which tools they should be familiar with (e.g., the calendar) and which tools they are responsible for completing (e.g., skills monitor). The following are samples and descriptions of tools that should be reviewed with preceptors.

Skills Monitors

Although skills will vary from institution to institution or unit to unit, the design of the tool need not vary (see Table 4-3). The skills monitor should have directions, a space for self-assessment, a rating scale, and a sign-off mechanism. A performance standard is also recommended to indicate the level of expertise that the orientee must achieve by the end of the orientation or probationary period. The preceptor should understand that not all experiences will be available or that it may not be possible to achieve mastery of all skills.

TABLE 4-3   Skills Monitor

Medical Surgical RN Skills Monitor

Name:_____   Unit:_____

Information: This inventory of required nursing skills shall be completed by the end of your probation. You are responsible for having your preceptor or clinical instructor sign off on each skill after you demonstrate competency. Keep this document current and present it to the Clinical Coordinator for evaluation purposes. After probation, this document will become a part of your record.

Directions: 1. Read each competency and select a code from the following list which best describes your knowledge and/or experience. Put the code number you select in the column labeled "Self Assessment".

Performance Code
1. No experience
2. Perform with assistance
3. Perform under supervision
4. Perform independently
N/A   Not applicable to unit and/or site

2. Each time you demonstrate a skill have the preceptor or clinical instructor initial and date a code number that best describes your skill level. You are expected to reach the performance standard for most of the competencies by the end of probation. Your Clinical Coordinator will review this check-list with you throughout the orientation and probationary period.

COMPETENCY	Self Assessment Code #	Observer to initial & data under Code # 1 2 3 4				Perfor-mance standard
I. Assessment: A. Measures patient's vital signs: 1. TPR						4
2. Blood Pressure						4
3. Neuro checks (Orientation to time, place person, response to directions and pain stimuli, pupillary reaction, extremity movement)						4
4. Height						4
5. Weight						4
6. CVP—set up, maintain, measure and record						2
II. Planning: A. Write initial plan of care —nursing diagnosis/need/focus/discharge planning and patient teaching needs						4
B. Establish goal with patient/family/SO						4
C. Write nursing interventions						4

continued

TABLE 4-3 *continued*

III. Implementation:							
A. Maintain respiratory function—							
1. Administration of oxygen—set up, initiate and administer:							
a. Nasal cannula							4
b. Face mask							4
c. Venti mask							4
d. Nonrebreathing mask							4
e. Trach collar							4
f. T-piece							4
2. Incentive spirometer —demonstrate use of							4
3. Coughing and deep breathing—demon-strate and work with patient							4
4. Scutining—lubricate catheter if applicable, insert, suction and withdraw							
a. Nasotracheal							3
b. Oropharyngeal							3
c. Nasopharyngeal							3
5. Tracheotomy care— perform tube care, clean wound, change dressing, document							3
6. Closed chest drainage—observe for leaks, maintain, measure output, assess and document respiratory status, assess dressing							

a. Gravity							3
b. Suction							3
7. Pulse oximeter— set-up, apply sensor, set alarms, reassure, interpret, record							3
8. Suction equipment— set-up and maintain							
a. Portable suction							4
b. Wall suction							4
9. Respiratory assist devices—set-up and maintain							
a. Nasal CPAP for sleep apnea							2
b. Nocturnal positive pressure ventilation via nasal mask							2
c. Negative pressure ventilation (pneumosuit)							2
10. Ventilator management—identify F_{O_2} rate, TV mode. Respond, reset and interpret alarms. Check humidification source and vent temperature. Empty excess water from tubing and administer nebulized medication							2
B. Maintain cardiovascular function							
1. Code management—							

continued

TABLE 4-3 *continued*

a. Verbalize emergency number to call					4
b. Initiate and administer BCLS					4
c. Bring code cart and EKG machine					4
d. Attach O2 to ambu bag					4
e. prepare suction machine					4
f. prepare code medications					4
2. Code cart and equipment maintenance—check cart, check O2 tank, check suction and EKG machine					4
3. Blood products: a. Check, administer and document blood product administration					3
b. Monitor patient during administration					3
c. State policy/ procedure to use with transfusion reaction					3
C. Support and maintain nutritional requirements— 1. TPN, PPN, Intralipids—					

administer and document							4
2. Tube feeding—check for placement, administer feedings, check and record residual							
a. Nasogastric							4
b. Gastrostomy							3
c. Jejunostomy							3
3. Intravenous therapy (peripheral, intermittent infusion devices)							
a. Verify order							4
b. Insert line/device and label dressing							4
c. Label bag and tubing							4
d. Calculate and regulate rate							4
e. Flush intermittent infusion device							4
f. Assess and document site condition							4
4. Central line/Peripherally inserted central line catheter care							
a. Assess, change dressing, document site condition							4
b. Access central venous access catheter with subcutaneous reservoir							3

continued

TABLE 4-3 *continued*

c. Flush/ heparinize as per policy/ procedure or as ordered by MD						3
D. Administer medications: 1. Oral						4
2. Nasogastric						4
3. Subcutaneous						4
4. Intramuscular						4
5. Intravenous via peripheral line, intermittent infusion device, central line						4
6. Rectal						4
7. Vaginal						4
8. Ophthalmic						4
9. Otic						4
10. Topical						4
11. PCA						4
12. Nebulization (CPN)						4
E. Care for patient with limited mobility— 1. Decubitis ulcer management—assess risk factors, document stage/observation, initiate and maintain skin care protocol						4
2. Range of motion exercises—initiate and maintain skin care protocol						4
3. Protective positioning and turning						4

4. Transfer to chair						4
5. Transfer to stretcher						4
6. Ambulation						
a. With assistance						4
b. Cane						3
c. Crutches						3
d. Walker						3
7. Care of Patient with immobilizing device						
a. Cast						3
b. Traction						3
c. Sling						3
F. Maintain elimination function of GI and GU systems						
1. Care of the patient with naso-gastric tube—check for placement, and patency maintain suction, check bowel sounds, perform nasal care and document						4
2. Enemas						
a. Fleets						4
b. TWE						4
c. Retention						4
3. Colostomy care—						
a. Skin care						4
b. Observation of stoma						4
c. Application of appliance						4
d. Irrigation (with cone only)						3

continued

TABLE 4-3 *continued*

4. Catheterization— insert, maintain, record output, provide perineal care, remove a. Indwelling						4
b. Straight						4
5. Suprapubic catheter care						3
6. External catheter (condom)						4
7. Peritoneal dialysis— a. Initiate peritoneal dialysis						3
b. Add medications						3
c. Perform solution exchange						3
d. Obtain dialysate culture and cell count						3
e. Perform catheter and exit site care						3
f. Terminate peritonaeal dialysis						3
G. Collect specimens 1. Guaiac testing						4
2. Urine for urinalysis						4
3. Urine for culture and sensitivity a. Indwelling						4
b. Clean catch						4
4. 24 hour urine collection						4
5. Urine for S & A's						4
6. Wound for C & S						4
7. Sputum for C & S						4
8. Sputum for AFB						4
9. Blood glucose monitoring						4

H. Implement principles of infection control						
1. Handwashing						4
2. CDC isolation categories						4
3. Universal precautions						4
4. Sterile dressing changes						4
5. Gowning, gloving, masking						4
6. Disposal of contaminated linen/ trash						4
7. Handling of reusable equipment						4
8. Use of particulate respirators						4
I. Maintain patient, visitor, staff safety, environmental safety—						
1. Falls prevention— identify patient at risk, initiate and maintain patient safety alert protocol						4
2. Restraints—identify need, assess and provide comfort measures, renew order, document						4
3. Fall safe device— initiate, maintain and monitor						4
J. Identify patient precautions (suicidal and non-suicidal)— initiate, maintain and document						4

continued

TABLE 4-3 *continued*

K. Miscellaneous						
1. Applies						
a. Abdominal binder						4
b. Elastic stockings, Ace bandages—observe peripheral circulation including color, sensation, capillary refill, skin temperature, peripheral pulse.						4
2. Utilize equipment—set up, initiate and monitor						
a. Hypo/hyper-thermia blanket						4
b. Bedscale/chair scale						4
c. Electronic thermometer						4
d. Heating pad						4
e. Air mattress						4
f. Therapeutic bed						4
g. Infusion pump/controller						4
h. Kangaroo pump						4
i. Continuous Passive Motion (CPM) device						3
j. Hoyer lift						3
k. Sequential Compression device						3
3. Maintain drains						
a. Jackson Pratt						3
b. Hemovac						3
4. Post-mortem care						3

L. Document patient care—							
1. Admission nursing assessment							4
2. Patient care plan/ MPC							4
3. Activity Flow Record							4
4. Nursing Treatment Kardex/MPC							4
5. Fluid Balance Record							4
6. Medication Administration Record (MAR)							4
7. Integrated Progress Notes							4
8. Pre-op checklist							4
9. Pre/Post operative Teaching Record							4
10. Informed consent							4
11. Transfer summary							4
12. Restraint flow sheet							4
13. Discharge nursing assessment							4
14. Patient discharge instructions							4
15. PCA Administration Record							4
16. Peritoneal dialysis flowsheet							3
17. Fingerstick accession quality control form							4
18. Pressure Ulcer Risk Assessment/ Flowsheet							4
19. Medicus Classification							4

continued

TABLE 4-3 *continued*

IV. Other (unit specific)						

Although the following are not strictly just skills, you are expected to complete the following and be independent upon completion of orientation:

COMPETENCY	Self Assessment Code #	Observer to initial & data under Code #				Performance standard
		1	2	3	4	
I. Admission (obtain report, prepare patient area, perform assessment, complete data base, transcribe MD orders, write care plan and kardex/ MPC)						4
II. Intershift Report (give systematic assessment, needs and problems identified, interdisciplinary intention and care administered)						4

III.	Transfer (accept and send patients, write and give verbal report)						4
IV.	Discharge (confirm discharge arrangements, complete discharge teaching, complete discharge summary and discharge instructions)						4
V.	Patient Teaching (identify learning needs, provide and document teaching)						3
VI.	Time Management (organize and prioritize patient care assignment, delegate appropriately)						3
VII.	Charge Nurse. 1. Assess patients' needs and skills levels of staff						3
	2. Write and communicate staff's patient assignment, delegated tasks, scheduled meetings and inservice classes.						3
	3. Assess and follow-up Unit Secretary's performance of clerical and receptionists' responsibilities.						3
	4. Orient floats to unit routine.						4
	5. Inform nursing office of unit staffing issues.						3

continued

TABLE 4-3 *continued*

6. Obtain periodic update of patient care needs/ unit management issues form nursing staff. Communicate/ facilitate communica- tion of patient care/ unit management issues to appropriate physician, and designated supervisor (cc or covering CC. ACN. DN)						3

Initials/Signatures/Title

Orientation Clinical Summary:

_____

_____

_____

_____

_____

_____

Signatures:

Instructor: _____ Date: _____

Clinical Coordinator: _____ Date: _____

Preceptor: _____ Date: _____

Orientee: _____ Date: _____

Scheduling

It is ideal if the orientee has all clinical days with the same preceptor. This minimizes the distress orientee's experience when
bounced from preceptor to preceptor. Providing the preceptor
with a calendar of the orientee's schedule enables the preceptor to
plan her activities to best meet the needs of the orientee. If needed,
orientees can be scheduled to work weekends with their preceptor.
Although instructor support is not usually available on the
weekends, the consistency of maintaining the link to the preceptor
usually outweighs this drawback. If the orientee has been hired for
an evening or night shift, arrangements can be made to have a preceptor on the assigned shift. However, it is usually recommended
that the orientee begin clinical orientation on the day shift when
the supervision and support of the nurse manager and the instructor are more available. Transition to the assigned shift can be based
on the progress observed in this first phase of orientation.

The greater the flexibility of the orientation program, the more
complex the calendar can become. If, for example all classes are
rigidly scheduled at the same time each month, the calendar is a
simple affair. On the other hand, if self-instructional materials are
used in the orientation program and learners progress at substantially different speeds, covering a variety of topics at different
times, the calendar can become a nightmare. There are ways, however, to simplify the orientee's calendar without eliminating the
flexibility. For example, one can have the preceptor, orientee, and
instructor work on the calendar together. This involves the participants and makes them feel in control of the orientation process
and allows them to make necessary changes.

Guidelines

Providing preceptors with guidelines helps the preceptor in planning the clinical experience for the orientee (see Table 4-4).
Guidelines should give the preceptor an idea of how the average
protégé should be progressing. For example, guidelines may indicate that orientees should begin administering medications during
their second week of orientation after they have completed the
learning activities on medication administration. With this concept

TABLE 4-4   GENERAL ORIENTATION: Suggested Clinical Assignments:
Medical/Surgical Specialty

Orientation	Orientation Content	Suggested Patient Categories/Needs	Suggested Clinical Activities

Week #1	1. Concepts of Adult Learning
	2. Review of Skills Monitor
	3. Personnel Policies
	4. Intake and Output
	5. TPN/pump
	6. Fire Safety
	7. Comprehensive Nursing Documentation
	8. Respiratory Therapy
	9. Medication Transcription Documentation and Administration
	10. Patient Teaching
		Patient Admission
		Patient requiring IV fluids
			*No transcription of orders or medication administration
			
			Day #1
			1. Shadow preceptor and observe both unit and patient care routines
			2. Complete Scavenger Hunt
			3. Select 2 patients assigned to preceptor and review:
			  a) patient chart/care plan
			  b) nursing treatment kardex
			  c) medication administration record
			
			Day #2
			1. Deliver care to selected patients with instructor/preceptor support.

continued

TABLE 4-4   *continued*

Week #2	1. General Transcription 2. Blood and Blood Products Administration 3. Infection control 4. Skin Care 5. Emergency Management 6. Alternate Level of Care (ALC) 7. Central Venous Access	1. Patients receiving Respiratory Therapy 2. Patient requiring skin care 3. Pre-operative patient 4. Patient requiring teaching 5. Patient requiring TPN	*No transcription of orders. Patient care assignment of 2–4 patients with preceptor/instructor support. 1. Deliver total care to assigned patients including: a) physical care b) teaching c) documentation d) medication administration following supervised experience 2. Participate in rounds/report 3. Attend Multidisciplinary Rounds
Week #3	1. Legal Aspects of Nursing 2. Patient Observation Precautions 3. Safety Policies/ Procedures: a) Environmental b) External disaster c) Radiation d) Body Mechnics	1. Patient requiring isolation 2. Patient requiring blood transfusion 3. Patient classified in ALC category 4. Post operative patient 5. Patient Discharge 6. Patient with Central Venous Access Device	Patient care assignment of 3–5 patients with preceptor/ instructor support 1. Deliver total care to assigned patients including: a) physical care b) Medication administration

continued

			c) transcription of orders
			d) patient teaching
			e) documentation
			2. Participate in rounds/report
			3. Check emergency cart independently

Week #4	1. Resource People
	2. AIDS Center Program
	3. Medicus Classification System
	4. Quality Assurance/ Improvement
		1. Patient care experiences not completed in Weeks #2 and #3	Patient care assignment of 4–6 patients with preceptor/ instructor support
			1. Deliver total care to assigned patients including:
			  a) physical care
			  b) medication administration
			  c) transcription of orders
			  d) patient teaching
			  e) documentation
			2. Participate in rounds/report
			3. Complete Medicus Classification on assigned patients

of the "average" orientation, preceptors will be able to pace themselves and their orientees appropriately.

Resource Materials

Preceptors find it helpful if they are aware of available resource materials to use with their orientee. Policy and procedure manuals are immediately available on the patient care unit. In addition, preceptors should review for themselves and their orientees other pertinent materials. Reference manuals, computer reference materials, textbooks, patient education materials, and closed-circuit television broadcasts are a few samples of materials to which they could refer the orientee. In addition, the instructor may want to make the preceptor aware of educational materials, such as learning packages, videos, or other materials.

Program Format

The format of a Preceptor Training Program will depend on the amount of time allocated for the training. Content could be covered in a cursory manner in a half day, or reviewed in detail with experiential exercises in a two-day program. A cost-benefit analysis can be used in determining the length of the program. One should be able to justify the amount of time and money expended on preceptor training according to the benefits accrued as a direct result of the program. For example, including a cultural diversity component of two hours in length might be justified as an investment in preventing the loss of an orientee due to cultural pressures. However, conducting a two-day training program in an institution of cultural homogeniety would clearly be a mistake.

Frequently, the most convenient, cost-effective, and educationally feasible amount of time for preceptor training is a one-day program. A one-day program can be designed in a workshop model, which allows time in the morning for presenting and discussing key elements, and time in the afternoon for exercises, questions and answers, and group problem-solving. Prior to the program, preceptor candidates should receive selected readings to review in preparation for the course. This assures that all participants have a minimum baseline of information. It also gives preceptors an opportunity to test their independent learning skills and reminds them, in some small way, of the information overload that orientees experience.

It is the role of the Preceptor Training Program faculty to review, reinforce, and clarify learning. Using real-life case studies (ideally contributed by preceptors from within the institution) as starting points, the faculty can help the preceptors identify the principles that should guide their practice as a preceptor. Rather than lecture style, the class format should be designed as a discussion or seminar. As a method of evaluation, a workshop element can be incorporated at the end of the program.

In the workshop, preceptors can be divided into groups and presented with orientation training scenarios. Using the concepts they learned during the program, the preceptor groups attempt to "solve" these scenarios. At the end of the workshop, each preceptor group presents its solution to the class. This workshop assures the faculty that the preceptors understand the principles of adult education and their responsibilities as preceptors. The workshop also utilizes a collaborative problem solving approach that can be used in the clinical setting.

If time allows, role playing these sessions can be included in the preceptor training. If there is hesitation among the group to engage in role-playing, an alternative is using videotaped role-plays, done by the faculty or former preceptors. Program participants can then critique the role play and suggest or demonstrate alternative approaches.

For institutions where preceptor enrollment is small and/or instructor resource limited, the content of the Preceptor Training Program can be put into an independent study format using videoprograms, written reference materials, and self-assessment tools. Although this model is not ideal, because it lacks the interaction found in a group training activity, it is adequate for providing preceptors with a beginning conception of their role. Its limitation is somewhat mitigated by the timeliness with which preceptor training can be delivered. There is no need for a staff member to wait several months for the next Preceptor Training Program, since the self-instructional training can occur at any time. If a self-instructional model is selected for preceptor training, it can be supplemented with shorter, 2-hour workshops in which preceptors who have completed the self-instructional training can come together to discuss questions, problems, or concerns that they are experiencing in their role as a preceptor. This workshop would provide reinforcement and clarification of the role of the preceptor, and also provide the group support that may have been missed by the preceptors in their initial training.

Preceptor Program Supports

Ideally, orientation is seen as a responsibility of all employees, not just the members of the education department. With the participation of peers, orientation becomes more than just a classroom exercise. Peer participation can transform orientation into a dynamic, meaningful, learning experience. To support peer participation in orientation, job descriptions should be written to include the responsibility each staff member has in orienting a new staff member. At a minimum, a staff member should be able to assist in some way in the transition of the "new kid on the block" into a colleague who can pull his own weight. Preceptors take this expectation one step further. After receiving training, they are capable of providing a professional clinical orientation for the new nurse.

Internal motivating factors, usually the desire and satisfaction related to teaching, contribute greatly to the staff person's willingness to precept a new nurse. However, external motivators and rewards can make the role that much more appealing.

Any one or a combination of the following strategies can be used to communicate to the preceptor that the institution recognizes and acknowleges their commitment.

- Offering continuing education credits for attending the Preceptor Training Program;
- Presenting preceptors with a certificate and a pin;
- Providing salary differential for precepting;
- Publishing preceptors' names and pictures in the hospital newsletter; and
- Sending preceptors a letter of recognition from nursing leadership.

Recognition of preceptors should not be considered a "one-shot deal" as the preceptor role is one that requires daily commitment and can sometimes feel like a thankless task. A bad experience with one orientee can leave a preceptor feeling dejected and can erase any memories of the pluses originally associated with the role. Preceptors should be prepared for these bad times in their initial training. Such problems as mismatches between orientee and preceptor, orientee termination due to performance problems, or a variety of other pressures involved in being a preceptor should be discussed in the training program. In addition, ongoing support and recognition can help to alleviate preceptor burnout. These supports could include:

- professional journal subscriptions;
- annual Preceptor Recognition Reception;
- opportunity to participate in additional continuing education activities;
- instructor feedback on preceptor skills;
- nurse manager feedback on preceptor involvement; and
- orientee evaluation of preceptor's role in orientation.

Supports like the ones listed above indicate to the preceptor that the institution is willing to support ongoing development in the preceptor role.

THE PRECEPTOR ROLE IN ACTION

Assignment Planning for the Orientee

There are three components involved in planning a clinical assignment for the orientee:

1. Reviewing the orientee's self-assessment form;
2. Providing observational experiences for the orientee; and
3. Planning the patient-care assignment.

The first or fundamental component of planning the orientee's clinical assignment is the preceptor's review of the orientee's self-assessment. Before the first clinical experience, the orientee usually completes some version of an assessment tool. The protégé is then directed to share this information with the preceptor. The preceptor reviews this tool, taking into consideration the orientee's educational background and past work experience. The assessment tool provides the preceptor with a concrete starting point related to the orientee's technical skills when selecting patient-care assignments.

The second component of assignment planning involves providing observational experiences for the orientee. Depending on the orientee's past experience, the time devoted to observational experiences will vary. Observational experiences would include activities such as shadowing the preceptor for the purpose of observing unit routines, patient-care activities, time management, and priority setting. An experienced nurse is usually ready for a modified independent patient care assignment after one day of observing the preceptor. However, a new graduate might need additional observational time due to the sensory overload of the orientation.

Additional observational experiences can be designed to meet the needs of the orientee. For example, an operating room observational experience may help an orientee on a surgical unit to do better pre-op teaching. The preceptor should be given latitude in determining the necessary observational experiences, keeping in mind the limited time of orientation.

The third component of assignment planning is the actual patient-care assignment. The orientee's patient assignment is made by the preceptor, if possible, with input from the orientee. This collaborative approach works well not only at the beginning of orientation, but long after orientation, when preceptor and orientee are true peers. In addition to using the skills monitor data to determine the assignment, the preceptor is encouraged to take into consideration the orientee's comfort level during the observational experience. If, for example, the orientee demonstrated extreme nervousness when talking with patients or staff members, the preceptor should start with an easier patient care assignment, graduating the acuity of the patients with increasing orientee confidence. For the inexperienced orientee, the preceptor might initially choose to share his/her assignment with the orientee. The two would work together in a "buddy system" and the preceptor would delegate aspects of patient care to the orientee. The preceptor would be right beside the inexperienced orientee as an "on the spot" resource and support. On the other hand, an experienced nurse whose questions and comments during the observational experience indicate a high-level knowledge and confidence might work independently from the start using the preceptor as a resource.

Even with the best of planning, relevant patient care experiences may be difficult to provide. A specific patient care experience may not be available within the preceptor's assignment or in the clinical setting. Even if it involves shifting to a different location, arrangements should be made for the orientee to be assigned to a patient who provides the learning opportunity, ideally with the preceptor also covering the patient. This is preferable to the orientee being split between two preceptors. It is important for the preceptor to be committed to providing the orientee with as many experiences as feasible during the dedicated time of orientation when support and guidance are readily available.

When a relevant patient care experience is not available in the clinical setting during orientation, other options are available. For example, the orientation period could be extended or a plan could be made to provide the experience after the orientation period. In the later situation the orientee and the nurse manager need to mutually agree to seek out the experience when the opportunity presents itself.

Evaluating the Orientee

From the onset of orientation, the orientee shares responsibility for assessing learning needs, identifying and utilizing resources, and requesting specific patient-care assignments that validate the orientee's competency. The preceptor, nurse educator, and nurse manager respect the orientee's input and make available tools, guidelines, and resources to enable the orientee to succeed.

At the conclusion of orientation, the orientee should complete a summative self-evaluation. This summative evaluation tool could be the self-assessment tool used at the start of the orientation or could be the performance evaluation tool based on the job description. This summative evaluation is an opportunity for the orientee to note progress, problems, or concerns prior to assuming full staff responsibility. If the orientation has been successful, this summative self-evaluation is usually a satisfying experience for the orientee. If the orientation was problematic, the final self-evaluation is an opportunity for the orientee to identify specific weaknesses and discuss them with the nurse manager.

For some orientees self-evaluation is an intimidating and difficult process, however, it is an important skill that nurses will use on an ongoing basis during their careers. If care was taken during the initial self-assessment to make it a positive, nonthreatening situation, the summative self-assessment will be less intimidating. Orientees will have little temptation to give a falsely high or low rating of their skills if a nonpunitive approach is taken to skills assessment throughout orientation.

The orientee's self-assessment provides the starting point for the collaborative evaluation completed by the nurse manager, preceptor, and nursing instructor. Throughout the orientation the preceptor communicates with the nurse manager and nurse educator providing updates on the orientee's progress. These update sessions should be conducted on a regularly scheduled basis, or as daily informal "on-the-go" communications. Based on these updates, the orientation plans can be revised and made more responsive to the needs of the orientee.

Final Written Evaluation

The final assessment of the orientee, completed by the nurse manager, preceptor, and nurse educator, should reflect the orientee's competency on completion of orientation. Early anecdotal findings need not be included in the final evaluation if the orientee has demonstrated a sustained improvement. The written evaluation should be discussed by all involved with the orientee. There should be no surprises in this session for the orientee if communication has been open and consistent during the orientation period. The final evaluation can be an opportunity for all participants to reflect on the achievements and obstacles encountered during the orientation.

Addressing the situation of the orientee who has been unable to meet the performance expectations is always stressful. Preceptors need the support of both the nurse manager and the nurse educator when this occurs. Preceptors can feel guilty, frustrated, angry, disheartened, or experience a combination of all these emotions. In situations of this type, substantial efforts need to be devoted by all involved with orientation. Although this can be exhausting, such outcomes are the exception rather than the rule; failure to address the situation carefully can have personal, professional, and organizational repercussions. Additional support may be sought from supervisory, administrative, and legal staff. Handling a poor performance situation should always be a team effort with the orientee being involved and informed on a regular basis.

If the orientee has been successful, this can be a time to enjoy the positive feedback and provide an opportunity for future planning. The orientee's success can predispose his/her to consider further educational pursuits, professional development activities, or involvement in unit projects. This is also an excellent opportunity to plant the "seed" for preceptoring in the orientee that may later develop into a willingness and desire to become a preceptor. One suggestion is to have the orientees write personal descriptions of their orientation and their goals for the future and place these notes in sealed, self-addressed envelopes. These "letters," which can be mailed back to the orientees at a date specified in the future (i.e., six months, one year, on acceptance as a preceptor) are an excellent way to maintain a sensitivity to new staff members long after the feeling of "newness" has faded.

Evaluating the Preceptor

As for all staff members, the preceptor is evaluated at regular intervals, usually on an annual basis. A part of this annual performance evaluation should include a review of the nurse's willingness and ability to precept new staff members. If the job description includes this precepting expectation, then it should be reflected in the performance evaluation tool, and there will be no surprises when the nurse is evaluated on precepting abilities.

This formal evaluation is important in validating the value and importance of the preceptor role, but it is not always timely in giving the preceptor the feedback that is needed immediately after orienting a new staff member. An evaluation process that parallels the orientee's evaluation process should be implemented. Throughout the orientation, the preceptor should be given feedback on his or her performance in the role. The "on-the-go" meetings with the nurse manager and the nurse educator should include observations and suggestions on the preceptor's abilities, as well as, the orientee's progress. At the end of each precepting experience, the preceptor should have the opportunity to discuss his or her precepting skills with the nurse educator and the nurse manager. The preceptor should be given an opportunity for self-assessment prior to receiving the feedback. This will encourage and strengthen the preceptor's ability for self-evaluation and will give the preceptor insight into the process of self-evaluation in which the orientee participates.

The orientee's evaluation of orientation may include specific comments regarding the preceptor. These comments can be shared with the preceptor, but care should be taken to do this in a positive manner. Any unfavorable comments could cause the preceptor to become angry or hurt. The nurse educator should be able to relay the comments to the preceptor with an eye to improving future orientations, rather than blaming the preceptor for errors in the past.

SUMMARY

This chapter reviewed the design and implementation of a preceptorship program for nurse orientees in a health care center. It is recommended that before initiating a preceptor program that an assessment of the current needs and capabilities of the institution, the nursing department, and the incumbent staff be conducted. This will assure a preceptor program that is appropriate for the institution and in congruence with its mission and goals.

Important components of a preceptor program include: criteria for preceptor selection, definition of preceptor responsibilities, program curriculum, orientation tools, and preceptor evaluation. To conduct an effective preceptor program, it is essential to use educational strategies that are consistent with the principles of adult education.

REFERENCES

Andersen, S. (1991). Preceptor teaching strategies: Behaviors that facilitate role transition in senior nursing students. *Journal of Nursing Staff Development, 7(4),* 171–175.

Benner, P. (1984). *From novice to expert.* Menlo Park, CA: Addison-Wesley.

Brookfield, S. (1990). *Understanding and facilitating adult learning.* San Francisco: Jossey-Bass.

Duff, M., & Kirsivali-Farmer, K. (1994). The challenge: Developing a preceptorship program in the midst of organizational change. *The Journal of Continuing Education, 25(3),* 115–119.

Gregorc, A. F. (1984). *Gregorc style delineator: Development, technical, and administration manual.* Maynard, MA: Gabriel Systems.

Hartline, C. (1993). Preceptor selection and evaluation: A tool for educators and managers. *Journal of Nursing Staff Development, 9(4),* 188–192.

Honey, P., & Mumford, A. (1989). *Capitalizing on your learning style.* King of Prussia, PA: Organizational Design and Development.

Kolb, D. A. (1993). *Learning style inventory user's guide.* Boston: McBer Training Resource Group.

Meng, A., & Conti, A. (1995). Preceptor development: An opportunity to stimulate critical thinking. *Journal of Nursing Staff Development, 11(2),* 71–76.

Merriam, S., & Cafferarella, R. (1991). *Learning in adulthood.* San Francisco: Jossey-Bass.

Mulqueen, J. (1995). *Facilitating adults' adjustment to college: A manual for faculty.* Unpublished manuscript.

Schwerin, J., Gaster, K., Krolinkowski, J., & Sherman-Justice, D. (1994). Staff nurse leadership and professional growth in the mentor role. *Journal of Nursing Staff Development, 10(3),* 139–144.

Chapter **5**

BEYOND PRECEPTORSHIP: INTERNSHIPS AND EXTERNSHIPS, FELLOWSHIPS/ APPRENTICESHIPS, AND MENTORSHIPS

Anne E. Belcher, PhD, RN, FAAN

There is a wide variety of educational/orientation programs available to students, new graduate nurses, and experienced nurses in practice. These programs include, but are not limited to internships, externships, fellowships, and apprenticeships. The general purposes of these programs are (a) to bridge the gap between academic preparation and initial clinical practice, while easing role transition; (b) to improve the recruitment, retention, and job satisfaction of nurses in health-care agencies; and (c) to produce a positive cost-benefit ratio in the recruitment/orientation/retention process. In addition, mentorship offers unique opportunities for continuing professional development to both mentor and protégé.

This chapter will:

- describe the similarities and differences among internships, externships, fellowships/apprenticeships, and mentorship (see Table 5-1);
- identify the individual and organizational benefits of these types of programs; and
- identify potential areas for research.

TABLE 5-1   Comparisons of Various Educational/Orientation Programs

Characteristics	Internships	Externships	Apprenticeships/Fellowships	Mentorships
1. Arrangement	Formal	Formal	Formal	Informal
2. Goals	Build consistent decision-making skills. Promote adaptation to work environment. Support development of competent practitioners. Improve recruitment and retention	Provide semi-structured work experience for nursing students.	Opportunity to work on a particular project for an organization or institution.	Teach protégés specific skills. Develop protégé's intellectual capabilities. Guide protégé's entry into and advancement within professional/organization. Serve as exemplar for the protégé.
3. Type of instruction	Includes didactic/clinical component	Conferences/clinical	Individual guidance	Individual guidance

4.	Length of time	8 weeks to one year	Short term: depends on student's schedule	Varies, depending on project	Indefinite; may extend over many years.
5.	Relationship	One-to-one	One-to-one	Usually one-to-one	One-to-one
6.	Reimbursement	To the "protégé"	To the extern	To the apprentice/fellow if available	None
7.	Advantages	Fewer absences from work. Lower attrition rate. Improved clinical competency. Improved integration into the work setting	Practical "real-life" experience gained	Opportunity to work with experts in a specific field/profession	Positive impact on professional growth. Increased satisfaction with the profession.

121

Each type of educational/orientation program has entrance/ selection requirements, a curriculum, clinical experiences, and evaluation strategies. The agencies that offer one or more of these programs believe that they have a positive impact on the partici- pants' professional behaviors; values, attitudes, and beliefs about health care and nursing; job satisfaction; and participation in con- tinuing education. In the following sections, these programs will be described and potential areas for research suggested. In the final section of the chapter, mentorships will be considered.

INTERNSHIPS

Nursing internships, which were first developed and implement- ed in the early 1960s, are viewed as extended orientation programs intended to bridge the gap between the role of the student and that of the competent nurse (Schempp & Rompre, 1986).

An internship program is defined as a semi-structured, super- vised orientation, which includes didactic and clinical components (Ross, 1966). Sams, Baxter, and Palmer-Smith (1990) indicate that a professional internship should be based on the principle that all nurses must have at least entry-level competency in their special- ty before assuming full staff nurse function. They recommend the use of an adult learning approach, which includes identification of clinical competencies and interaction with preceptors.

The goals of nurse internships are (1) to build consistent deci- sion-making skills; (2) to promote adaptation to the work environment; and (3) to support the development of competent and proficient practitioners (Kopp et al., 1993). Many hospitals have implemented nurse internships in an effort to improve recruitment and retention of nursing staff based on the belief that they improve job satisfaction, lessen feelings of powerlessness, and decrease turnover rates. The use of concepts basic to professional nursing practice is deemed to be cost-effective as well. Sams, Baxter, and Palmer-Smith (1990) determined that such a program " (1) pro- vides administration with a means of defining entry-level practice according to national standards; (2) provides the manager with a validation mechanism that the nurse is able to practice all aspects of nursing, not just accomplish specific tasks; (3) provides the preceptors with a clear guide for directing clinical experiences; and (4) illustrates a specific set of professional criteria that enables nurses to collaborate with preceptors and to validate their abilities daily" (p. 94).

Ressler, Kruger, and Herb (1991) described a Critical Care Internship Program whose goals were: "to provide new graduate nurses with the opportunity to increase knowledge and acquire critical care nursing skills, to provide graduate nurses with a practical clinical experience under the supervision of an experienced nurse, and to increase the number of educated critical-care nurses available for employment" (p. 177). Classes presented included basic principles of critical-care nursing and a focus on how the principles could be applied to the clinical setting. The preceptor played a pivotal role in validating assessment skills, reinforcing application of knowledge at the bedside, and serving as a role model. Process and outcome evaluation strategies indicated that the Critical Care Internship Program provided the new graduate nurse with the knowledge and clinical experience needed to provide care for critically ill patients.

Craver and Sullivan (1985) found that new graduate nurses who participated in an internship program had fewer absences from work and a lower attrition rate than those new graduates who were not interns. However, no differences were found in job performance evaluations, job satisfaction, or nursing skills. Kopp and colleagues (1993) evaluated a Critical Care Nurse Internship Program (CCNIP) which provides didactic instruction and supervised clinical experience to graduate nurses seeking critical-care staff nurse positions. They determined that the CCNIP promoted clinical competency and assisted in the recruitment and retention of staff nurses in critical care. Rosenthal and Connors (1989) discovered that a collaborative Pediatric Intensive Care Unit/ Neonatal Intensive Care Unit (PICU/NICU) internship was a successful strategy for meeting the ongoing challenge of integrating the new graduate nurse into the critical care environment in a supportive and educationally sound manner. Cooney (1992) described a successful orientation program for new graduate nurses desiring work in obstetrics. The use of a Skills Check List, class days for didactic presentation of special topics, and an Orientation Evaluation

Scale, which measures the new employees' level of supervision needed, organization, precision, and understanding produced nurses who were prepared to meet professional standards of care, who were retained longer than in the past, and who valued ongoing participation in staff development.

Beth Israel Hospital in Boston has developed an internship program entitled Clinical Entry Nurse Residency Program for new graduate nurses. This standardized, two-year, planned first work experience provides graduates of baccalaureate or higher degree programs with the necessary skills and behaviors needed for fulfilling the professional nursing role. The program includes hands-on clinical teaching, ongoing mentorship, and career planning. The resident works with a clinical nurse sponsor, whose focus is on the process of "socialization" into professional nursing and individual career development.

The *objectives* of the residency are to:

- demonstrate the centrality of caring in professional nurse/patient/family relationships;
- demonstrate competence in providing quality, cost-effective nursing care;
- demonstrate leadership skills in all aspects of professional practice;
- formulate a plan for continued development and overall career goals; and
- appreciate the larger context of the health care delivery system.

Learning strategies include assigned readings, shadowing experiences, reading and writing clinical exemplars, presenting patients at rounds, reviewing research articles, attending committee meetings and lectures, and meeting with various resources in the institution (Duprat, 1995).

Internship programs represent an excellent opportunity for collaboration between nursing service and nursing education (Hartshorn, 1992). The program can be developed with school and hospital educators sharing responsibility for clinical and classroom experiences. Graduates' participation in the program might be arranged to enable them to earn academic credit. Hospital-based educators benefit by working with school of nursing faculty who have an in-depth understanding of the new graduate. School of nursing faculty benefit by working with hospital-based educators who are "up-to-date" regarding changes in the clinical setting.

Other factors that have been found to affect the success of an internship program include:

- program coordinator, faculty and preceptors who promote intern independence and staff involvement in all aspects of the program; and
- program content and format, which build upon rather than duplicate content and experience which interns had in their basic nursing program.

The suggested steps for designing, implementing, and evaluating an internship program are listed below (see Table 5-2). Several steps may be initiated at the same time. The first step is to appoint the program coordinator and faculty and to recruit staff nurses as preceptors. The second step is to develop the goals for the program, as well as specific intern objectives. These goals should be measurable and reflective of the expected competencies of the new employee, as well as the institutions' expected outcomes. The third step is to determine the length of the program. Program length may range from 6 weeks to 12 months and reflects the planners' assessment of the time needed to attain program goals and intern objectives. The fourth step is to design the implementation process, which includes (a) the determination of who will be eligible to apply (usually limited to new graduates); (b) development of an application form; (c) identification of other materials to be requested, such as a resume, goal statement, transcript and references; and (d) format of the entrance interview. Criteria for the selection of applicants should also be identified. The fifth step is curriculum design, which will include didactic and clinical components.

Most internship curricula focus on technical skills, assessment skills, documentation, time management, communication skills, and clinical decision-making ability. The sixth step is development of the evaluation plan, which has two components, one for interns and one for the program. The intern evaluation might include a

TABLE 5-2   Steps for Designing, Implementing, and Evaluating
Internship Programs

1. Appoint the program coordinator and faculty and recruit staff nurse preceptors.
2. Develop program goals and objectives.
3. Determine length of the program.
4. Design the implementation process that includes:
   - determination of eligibility criteria for candidates
   - development of application form
   - identification of other materials to be requested (e.g. resume, goal statement, transcript, references)
   - format for entrance interview.
   - criteria for selection of candidates
5. Design curriculum regarding:
   - technical skills
   - assessment skills
   - documentation
   - time management
   - communication skills
   - clinical decision making
6. Develop evaluation plan that includes outcome measures for:
   - intern skill development
   - performance appraisal
   - job satisfaction
   - work attendance and attrition
   - cost data analysis

skills test, clinical observation, staff evaluation, and self-evaluation components. The program evaluation might be developed to measure intern skill development, performance appraisal outcomes, job satisfaction, work attendance and attrition. Cost data should also be collected as justification for program benefit/continuation.

The issue of the interns' service commitment should also be addressed. Because interns usually receive full salary and benefits, the organization may require a written agreement for a specified period of employment.

During those years when there was a nursing shortage, nurse internships were developed to meet hospital, recruitment and retention needs. However, in recent years questions about the cost effectiveness of these programs as well as their actual impact on recruitment and retention have led hospitals to redesign or to eliminate such programs.

Kotecki (1992) completed an extensive review of the literature regarding internships since their inception in the 1960s and reached the following conclusion: "Many of the (Internship) programs are creative and innovative but, when compared with regular orientation programs, do not show significant differences in clinical ability, role transition, or recruitment. A relationship does seem to exist between internship programs and retention of graduate nurse employees" (p. 205). [For comparison, a regular orientation program is described in Chapter 4 of this book].

Most programs studied differed from standard orientation programs only in terms of their length. Kotecki (1992) suggested that different curricular designs, content, and experience might change the outcome of existing internship programs. On the other hand, the current health care economic climate may signal the demise of the internship program. Administrators might question the use of scarce resources for such programs when those resources could conceivably be better used to enhance the knowledge base and clinical competency of the employed nurse. In addition, the unanswered questions or conflicting answers to such questions as cost-benefit ratio, retention, job satisfaction, and clinical performance weaken arguments in favor of such programs.

Research Issues

The internship programs offer opportunities for research which to date have been lacking entirely or only descriptive. Research questions could and should be generated to address a variety of issues, such as the following:

- How should applicants be selected for these programs? What criteria should be used?
- How can articulation with schools of nursing be used to enhance new graduates' preparation for and faculty participation in these programs?
- What differences in curriculum design, content, and experiences are needed to assure the expected outcomes of such programs? How is the optimal length of such programs determined?
- What is the cost effectiveness of these programs? How is it measured? How are costs and benefits weighed to determine the value of the program?
- How do these programs effect recruitment and retention of staff? How is job satisfaction measured?
- How are preceptors best selected? How are they prepared, evaluated, and rewarded for their participation in these programs? How are they matched with potential interns?

More attention should be directed to the evaluation process as well. Many programs use subjective evaluation measures, which make it difficult to assess the actual benefit of the programs.

Some issues which might be addressed in the evaluation process are:

- What clinical performance evaluation tool is valid and reliable for determining nurses' success in these programs?
- How can preceptor, nurse manager and nurse/other health care professional colleague involvement and satisfaction with program participants be determined?

Externships

In general, an externship is a period of time during which a student works under the direction of someone with experience in the profession. A variety of terms have been used to describe such a structured work experience: field work, practicum, directed projects, and cooperative education. All have the common purpose of providing structured student experiences outside of the classroom (Konsky, 1976). According to Cottrell and Wagner (1990), it is in the externship that students apply what they have learned in school to a real life situation; it "provides a type of culminating experience to the education process" (p. 30). The *benefits* of an externship are as follows:

- Students attain the confidence and experience needed to handle successfully an entry-level position in the profession;
- Successful student externs may have an advantage in the job market over those who choose not to complete an externship;
- Professional contacts and networking opportunities can be invaluable to the extern when seeking an initial or future professional position.

The sponsoring educational institution gains personal contact with practicing professionals, contact which is important for public relations, for future student placement, and for opportunities to conduct applied field research. The externship site also benefits from student externs serving as additional staff to accomplish daily tasks and to initiate projects which may have been placed on the "back burner" due to inadequate employee time. Externs also offer fresh ideas and new insights to the sponsoring agency and its employees.

Constraints or problems presented by externships include such specific issues as inadequate supervision of the extern, as well as such comprehensive issues as lack of research on the development, administration, and effects of such a program on the extern and on the agency.

Nursing externships have been offered by schools of nursing and health-care agencies for many years. Most of these programs employ students during summers only and were designed to supplement nursing staff in the agency during those months when vacation coverage was needed. Many but not all nurse externs work for a salary which is usually equivalent to or somewhat higher than that of other nonlicensed personnel. Some hospitals provide special classes for the externs and use a preceptor model for clinical supervision. The employing agency anticipates that the externs will apply for a full-time position after they complete their nursing education. However, these programs are decreasing in number as hospitals "down-size" their registered nurse staff and employ more full-time unlicensed personnel.

Research Issues

Cottrell and Wagner (1990) raised some interesting questions regarding externship programs that are applicable to nursing:

- Are site visits made during the externship and, if so, who makes the visits?
- Can students receive salary and/or living expenses?
- Do formal procedures exist for the approval/certification of externship sites prior to student placement? What criteria are used in selecting externship sites?

Some of the questions raised by Cottrell and Wagner (1990) and others with regard to externships which are researchable include:

- How many nursing programs require their students to participate in externships?
- What differences are there between students who participate in externships and those who do not?
- If site visits are made, who conducts them and how are they calculated in a faculty members workload?
- Are there criteria which should be used in selecting internship sites for students?
- How is the student's performance in the externship evaluated and by whom?

While answers to all of these questions would be helpful, the last one posed could provide useful data to schools of nursing and to health-care settings interested in offering externship programs.

FELLOWSHIPS/APPRENTICESHIPS

Fellowships and apprenticeships provide the professional person with the opportunity to gain practical experience under the direction of another professional person. Fellowships and apprenticeships come, according to Buckalew (1984), "in all shapes and sizes—paid, unpaid—formal, informal—long, or short term" (p. 28). The fellow or apprentice agrees to work on a particular project for an organization, such as doing research or collecting data and, in turn, gains valuable knowledge and experience while working with experts in the specific field.

Buckalew (1984) has the following suggestions for a nurse who is interested in pursing a fellowship or an apprenticeship:

- Have the name of an individual to contact or direct the inquiry to the personnel department.
- Identify your interest and background in the health-care system, not limiting your qualifications and experiences to nursing.
- Be prepared with a concise and updated resume; stress research completed, or in which you have participated; list all publications, including newspaper editorials.

Smaller councils within governmental agencies work on specific projects that may be of particular interest to the nurse applicant. Although these apprenticeships are usually unpaid and have small staffs and limited work space, they can be advantageous to the applicant if there are flexible work hours and the experience can be used for college credit or to help further a cause, for example, women's health, aging, or world hunger.

Agencies that offer fellowships/apprenticeships that may be available to interested and qualified nurses include:

- American Association for the Advancement of Retired Persons
- American Hospital Association
- American Nurses Association, including the Minority Fellowship Program

- Congressional Placement Office
- Department of Health and Human Services
- Health Care Finance Administration
- National Academy of Sciences
- White House Fellowships

State legislators and other nursing organizations may offer additional fellowships and apprenticeships. The focus of those listed above is on involvement in the political arena. As noted by Buckalew (1984):

Getting involved means work over and above the usual. It may demand sacrifice of time or money, in some cases both. However, the long-term benefits to the nursing profession will be worth it (p. 29).

MENTORSHIPS

Mentorship is a highly complex and developmentally important interpersonal relationship which may include, but is not limited to (a) teaching specific skills; (b) developing a protégé's intellectual capabilities; (c) intervening to assist in the protégé's entry into and advancement within the profession/organization; (d) providing advice, encouragement, and constructive criticism; (e) introducing the protégé to organizational operations, politics, and key players; and (f) serving as an exemplar who models the values and professionalism that the protégé can emulate. According to Bowen (1985), mentoring

. . . occurs when a senior person (the mentor) in terms of age and experience undertakes to provide information, advice, and emotional support for a junior person (the protégé) in a relationship lasting over an extended period of time and marked by substantial commitment by both parties. If the opportunity presents itself, the mentor also uses both formal and informal means of influence to further the career of the protégé (p. 31).

Yoder (1990) differentiates the concept of mentoring from those of role-modeling, sponsorship, precepting and peer strategizing. Role-modeling does not require a personal relationship between the model and the imitator. The model's role is a passive one, based on the assumption that the imitator will identify with the model and adopt the model's behaviors and values. Sponsorship has all of the characteristics of mentorship with the added aspect of finding the "right spot" for the protégé in the organization. Precepting has been previously defined in this book (see chapter 1). Peer strategizing usually consists of two persons who are peers in age and experience who engage in a reciprocal or mutual relationship which provides one of them with the needed guidance and assistance. This "trading of information" sustains the relationship over time.

The four stages of the mentor-protégé relationship are as follows:

Stage 1: Solicitation: This first stage involves the process of determining whether or not there is "good chemistry" between the mentor and protégé. During this time, the mentor is probing with the protégé around the thoughts and ideas they are both bringing to the relationship.

Stage 2: Inquiry: During this second stage, the mentor's primary function is to clarify expectations and define goals with the protégé. In this stage the protégé is often anxious with the mentor and has a feeling of being unable to meet expectations and goals.

Stage 3: Informational: This stage involves the protégé's knowledge and skill development including learning the ropes, gaining insight into the broader organizational experience, understanding the organizational game plan, and becoming familiar with who wields power.

Stage 4: Conversion: The fourth stage is symbolized by the protégé's autonomy and independence. The protégé, through the achievement of personal goals, begins to separate from the mentor. This stage may be characterized by disillusionment with the relationship, a simple parting of the ways, or a new and redefined relationship (Yoder, 1990).

Potential *dilemmas and barriers* of the mentor-protégé relationship were identified by May, Meleis, and Winstead-Fry (1982) as (a) independence versus protectiveness, in which the mentor may overprotect the protégé, thus stifling innovative ideas; (b) collegiality versus exploitation, in which the assertive and competitive protégé may cause the mentor to be too cooperative or the overly competitive mentor uses the protégé as a pawn to reach self-serving goals; (c) individuation versus protégé status, in which the mentors must encourage the protégé to be autonomous, not a clone of the mentor.

Darling (1984) categorizes mentors in such a way that each nurse can identify personal preferences and style with regard to this role. The four *mentor types* which she identifies are:

1. *The traditional mentor:* a person who is sufficiently experienced in a career to be able to give wise counsel to the protégé;
2. *The step-ahead mentor:* an older peer either in age or experience, one who can "pave the way," protect, or give valuable guidance to the younger person starting on the same path;
3. *The co-mentor:* a peer in age and experience who is engaged in a reciprocal or mutual relationship with the other person; the two either take turns providing guidance and assistance as it is needed or provide help to each other in specific areas; and
4. *The spouse mentor:* a special form of co-mentor who can be very significant in marriages; spouse mentoring can be either unilateral (with one person giving to another) or reciprocal (each providing guidance to the other in specific areas).

The type of mentor one tends to use is related to the stage of one's career life cycle.

The value of mentorship in nursing is its positive impact on the protégé's professional growth and the mentor's fulfillment in helping others to grow professionally. The challenge facing the new graduate nurse is to find a senior/experienced person or persons who will serve as a guide through his or her career.

Research Issues

There are numerous questions to be answered with regard to mentorship in nursing. Research is needed to address such issues as:

- value of multiple mentors as well as mentors outside nursing;
- effectiveness of a person in a supervisory position serving as a mentor;
- type of mentoring which fosters leadership development and scholarship; and
- differences between and relative benefits of male mentoring versus the feminist perspective on mentoring.

SUMMARY

Internships, externships, and apprenticeship/fellowships offer students and new graduates in nursing a variety of options for attaining professional competencies. The availability of and access to such opportunities is seriously threatened by the current health-care economic climate. The generation of partnerships between service and education, as well as more rigorous evaluation of existing programs, may be effective in gaining or sustaining support for such programs in the years to come.

Mentorship offers multiple benefits to the mentor, the protégé, and the profession. The nurse protégé who receives career advice, guidance, and promotion, role modeling, intellectual stimulation, and inspiration by a dedicated mentor will certainly be a more productive and exemplary professional nurse.

REFERENCES

Bowcd, D. (1985). Were men meant to mentor women? *Training and Development Journal, 39(1)*, 30–34.

Buckalew, J. (1984). Internships for nurses. *Home Healthcare Nurse, 2(4)*, 28–29.

Cooney, A. T. (1992). An orientation program for new graduate nurses: The basis of staff development and retention. *The Journal of Continuing Education in Nursing, 23(5),* 216–219.

Cottrell, R. R., & Wagner, D. I. (1990). Internships in community health education/promotion professional preparation programs. *Health Education, 21(1),* 30–33.

Craver, D. M., & Sullivan, P. P. (1985). Investigation of an internship program. *The Journal of Continuing Education in Nursing, 16(4),* 114–118.

Darling, L. A. (1984). Mentor types and life cycles. *The Journal of Nursing Administration, 14(11),* 43–44.

Duprat, L. (1994). The clinical entry nurse residency program. Offering bright futures for new graduate nurses. *Report on Professional Nursing at Boston's Beth Israel Hospital, 12 (2),* 1–3.

Hartshorn, J. C. (1992). Characteristics of critical care nursing internship programs. *Journal of Nursing Staff Development, 8(5),* 218–223.

Konsky, C. (1976). Practical guide to development and administration of an internship program: Issues, procedures, forms. *ERIC,* #ED 249 539, 1–30.

Kopp, M. E. A., Schell, K. A., Laskowski-Jones, L., & Morelli, P. K. (1993). Critical care internships: In theory and practice. *Critical Care Nurse, 12(8),* 115–118.

Kotecki, C. N. (1992). Nursing internships: Taking a second look. *The Journal of Continuing Education in Nursing, 23(5),* 201–205.

May, K. M., Meleis, A. I., & Winstead-Fry, P. (1982). Mentorship for scholarliness: Opportunities and dilemmas. *Nursing Outlook, 30(1),* 22–28.

Ressler, K. A., Kruger, N. R., & Herb, T. A. (1991). Evaluating a critical care internship program. *Dimensions of Critical Care Nursing, 10(3),* 176–184.

Rosenthal, C. H., & Connors, C. (1989). Pediatric/neonatal graduate nurse internship: A collaborative effort. *Pediatric Nursing, 15(2),* 194–196.

Ross, V. (1986). An internship for leadership in nursing. *Nursing Outlook, 14(2),* 40–42.

Sams, L., Baxter, K., & Palmer-Smith, P. (1990). A competency-based model for nurse internships. *Journal of Nursing Staff Development, 6(2),* 93–94.

Schempp, C., & Rompre, R. (1986). Transition programs for new graduates: how effective are they? *Journal of Nursing Staff Development, 2,* 150–156.

Yoder, L. (1990). Mentoring: A concept analysis. *Nursing Administration Quarterly, 15(1),* 9–19.

INDEX

SP *Springer Publishing Company*

TEACHING NURSING IN THE NEIGHBORHOODS
The Northeastern University Model

Peggy Matteson, RNC, PhD, Editor
Foreword by **Gloria Smith,** RN, PhD, FAAN

This volume describes a model of clinical education in which nursing students receive 50% of their clinical experiences in the community—often in settings where no other kind of health care services are available, like senior centers and day care centers. The program was developed as part of the Kellogg Foundation's Community Health Education, Research, and Service project, which fosters academic-community health care partnerships.

The book describes the issues confronting nurse educators in the face of a changing health care system, provides practical information on implementing community-based clinical experiences (including valuable appendixes of specific clinical activities), and evaluates how these students differ from traditionally trained students after graduation. Nurse educators will find ample information for adapting this program in their own schools.

Contents:

Springer Series: Teaching of Nursing
1995   256pp   0-8261-9100-2   *hardcover*

536 Broadway, New York, NY 10012-3955 • (212) 431-4370 • Fax (212) 941-7842

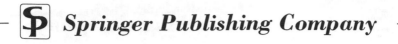 **Springer Publishing Company**

INCREASING PATIENT SATISFACTION
A Guide for Nurses

Roberta L. Messner, RNC, PhD, CPHQ
Susan J. Lewis, RN, PhD, CS

This manual guides nurses and others in the health care setting through the fundamentals of ensuring a satisfied "customer." It illustrates the many components of quality care, including how to provide clear and adequate information, create a hospitable environment, handle complaints efficiently, and design and utilize surveys of client satisfaction.

The authors draw from the principles of continuous quality improvement and other lessons learned from the business world, in addition to nursing's rich tradition of service. Written with warmth, sensitivity, and clarity, the book is an excellent resource for nursing students and practicing nurses. Health care institutions seeking good client relations will find this a suitable text for in-service training.

Contents:

What Do Patients Really Want? • The Changing American Healthcare Scene and Patient Satisfaction• Quality Isn't a Coincidence• Yes, Patients Do Have Rights • Patient Education: A Key to Increased Satisfaction • Creating a Hospitable and Healing Environment • How to Handle a Customer Complaint • Looking for the Lesson: Measuring/Evaluating Patient Satisfaction Findings • Be Kind to Yourself and Your Coworkers: A Plan for Enhanced Morale and Patient Satisfaction

1996   240pp   0-8261-9250-5   hardcover

536 Broadway, New York, NY 10012-3955 • (212) 431-4370 • Fax (212) 941-7842

℠ *Springer Publishing Company*

USING THE ARTS AND HUMANITIES TO TEACH NURSING
A Creative Approach

Theresa M. Valiga, EdD, RN
Elizabeth R. Bruderle, MSN, RN

This is a comprehensive sourcebook on using the humanities to teach nursing concepts. The authors, who have used the humanities to teach nursing at Villanova's College of Nursing since 1985, first give a general introduction to literature, television, film, and fine arts along with advantages and disadvantages of using each in nursing. They then describe selected nursing concepts, and provide specific examples of works of art that can be used to illustrate each.

> SPRINGER SERIES ON
> TEACHING OF NURSING
>
> **Using the Arts and Humanities to Teach Nursing**
> A Creative Approach
>
> THERESA M. VALIGA
> ELIZABETH R. BRUDERLE
>
> This comprehensive sourcebook is designed to help nurse educators be more creative in their teaching by using the humanities. The authors explain how the teaching of nursing may benefit from integrating elements of literature, television, film, and fine arts. The authors then describe selected nursing concepts along with specific examples of works of art that can be used to illustrate each concept.
> The numerous artworks discussed in the book include novels, short stories, children's literature, poetry, films, television, music, sculpture, paintings, opera, photography, and drama.
> This book can be used by faculty in any nursing education program—graduate, baccalaureate, associate degree, diploma, or LPN—and by staff development educators as well.
>
> SPRINGER PUBLISHING COMPANY ℠

These works include a variety of art forms — novels, short stories, children's literature, poetry, films, television, music, sculpture, paintings, opera, photography, and drama. The book is designed so that nurse educators can integrate this material into standard nursing courses, and it can be used by the faculty in graduate, baccalaureate, associate degree, diploma, LPN, or staff development education.

Springer Series on The Teaching of Nursing
1996   320pp   0-8261-9420-6   hardcover

536 Broadway, New York, NY 10012-3955 • (212) 431-4370 • Fax (212) 941-7842